Mastering Anxiety

The Nature and Treatment
of Anxious Conditions

W9-CSO-022

Mastering Anxiety

The Nature and Treatment
of Anxious Conditions

Ronald A. Kleinknecht, Ph.D.

Western Washington University
Bellingham, Washington

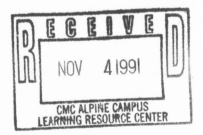

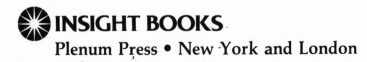

INSIGHT BOOKS

Plenum Press • New York and London

Library of Congress Cataloging-in-Publication Data

Kleinknecht, Ronald A. (Ronald Arthur)
    Mastering anxiety : the nature and treatment of anxious conditions
    Ronald A. Kleinknecht.
        p.   cm.
    "Insight book."
    Includes bibliographical references and index.
    ISBN 0-306-43769-4
    1. Anxiety. 2. Panic disorders.   I. Title.
    [DNLM: 1. Anxiety. 2. Aniety Disorders. 3. Anxiety Disorders-
-therapy.   WM 172 K64m]
    RC531.K544   1991
    616.85'223--dc20
    DNLM/DLC
    for Library of Congress   91-2218
                                                                   CIP

ISBN 0-306-43769-4

© 1991 Plenum Press, New York
A Division of Plenum Publishing Corporation
233 Spring Street, New York, N.Y. 10013

An Insight Book

Printed in the United States of America

Preface

Anxiety, fears, phobias, and panics are the most prevalent psychological disturbances in our society today. Greater than 12 percent of the adult population in the United States is so adversely affected by these emotions as to qualify for a psychiatric diagnosis of anxiety disorders. An additional 10 percent experience distressingly high levels of anxiety that interfere with their daily lives, although not severe enough to qualify for diagnosis. The vast majority of the remaining population, adults and children alike, frequently experience some form of fear or anxiety, if only on a milder or more transient basis. Clearly, anxiety and its disorders have personal meaning for everybody.

Although the conditions of anxiety and phobias have been observed and described for thousands of years, detailed analysis and scientific understanding of these conditions are of relatively recent origin. To a large extent, Sigmund Freud's writings and theories, at the turn of the century, stimulated the current interest in the causes and treatments of anxiety. Although new theories have replaced Freud's, it was from these early beginnings, and particularly over the past 30 years, that our understanding of fears, phobias, and anxiety has increased dramatically. Although we have made significant advances in understanding and treating anxiety-related disorders, much remains to be learned.

The purpose of this book is to provide a broad overview of this vast and important area of human emotion. In my survey, I describe the nature of anxiety as an emotion that sometimes serves us well whereas at other times, it imprisons us. My intention in this book is to facilitate an understanding of the nature of anxiety, the forms it takes when it becomes a problem, and the methods found effective in treating the problem. Although this book does not provide a prescription for self-treatment, it may help some people to understand the sources and forms that their anxiety has taken. If you find while reading that the illustrative case histories seem to match closely your own experiences, rest assured that you are in good company, as greater than 20 million others in the United States alone also fit these descriptions. Notable celebrities who have had anxiety disorders include Carly Simon (agoraphobia), John Madden (fear of flying), and Howard Hughes (obsessive-compulsive disorder).

In the first chapter, I review historical accounts and the linguistic roots of terms pertaining to anxiety, describe the core elements of anxiety, and briefly define the various conditions referred to as *anxiety disorders*. In the second chapter, I examine the biological and psychological roots of anxiety and then describe evolutionary and genetic contributions to anxiety in human beings and in animals, followed by a discussion of the psychological processes that build on the biological foundations. The psychological processes include classical conditioning and learning. Also described are the rudiments of Freud's theory and some current variants of existential theory pertaining to anxiety.

Chapter 3 begins with a presentation of the population prevalence of anxiety and anxiety disorders and how they vary by age and gender. The diagnostic process is discussed next and a variety of methods are presented that are used in measuring and assessing fears and anxiety states.

In Chapters 4, 5, and 6, I present detailed illustrations of the specific anxiety disorders. Chapter 4 contains my description of the simple or specific phobias—those intense fears of specific objects or situations—and the social phobias—those involving fear and anxiety associated with other individuals. In Chapter 5,

I deal with panic disorder and its frequent result, agoraphobia, the fear of going or being out alone. Chapter 6 begins with a description of posttraumatic stress disorder, in which I survey the anxiety condition that affects individuals who have been exposed to extraordinary traumas. Generalized anxiety disorder, the condition in which a person is constantly keyed up, always on edge, and chronically nervous, is also discussed in Chapter 6. The final condition to be illustrated in Chapter 6 is obsessive-compulsive disorder, in which uncontrollable thoughts and repetitive behavioral rituals seem to take charge of a person's mind and body.

Anxiety disorders of childhood are described in Chapter 7 and include over-anxious disorders, avoidant disorder, and separation anxiety disorder. Since the other anxiety disorders described in the preceding chapters can also occur in children, several childhood cases of these conditions are illustrated as well.

In the final three chapters, I describe treatments for the anxiety disorders. Chapter 8 focuses on several psychological treatment procedures that have proven highly effective in treating these anxiety conditions. In some instances, as with the simple phobias, these procedures can approach 100 percent effectiveness. Chapter 9 has several case studies in which the treatment procedures previously outlined are used to overcome the anxiety disorders. The final chapter I devote to a description of how psychiatric drugs work and list those drugs most commonly used in treating the anxiety disorders, along with their potential side effects.

All names and other identifying information concerning the illustrative cases have been fictionalized. Some examples are drawn from case studies that are published in professional journals, whereas others are composites of cases taken from my own research and treatment of anxiety disorders over the past 25 years.

R.A.K.

Contents

CHAPTER 1

An Introduction to Anxiety

Tom was home from another hectic day at work. He slumped into the easy chair. No matter how difficult it was, he knew he needed to relax. In a few minutes, the tenseness began to diminish. . . . He began to feel uneasy. Then, with a sudden start, he bolted fully upright in his chair! His heart was pounding so that he could actually see his chest pulsing and quivering. His clothes were becoming soaked with sweat; his throat felt like it was constricting. Was he dying? Having a heart attack? Losing his mind? He wanted to run, but to where? From what?

Cindy always carried cash; she never wrote checks or used credit cards. She knew how to use these modern conveniences, but she had an embarrassing problem: she could never sign a check in the presence of the cashier at the supermarket. The last time she tried, she ran crying from the store, leaving her groceries at the counter. She had panicked, her hand shook, she dripped sweat on the checkbook and smudged the ink. She "knew" she was going to make a spectacle of herself, and sure enough, the clerk noticed and asked her if something was wrong. It was then that her mind went blank and her knees went weak. It was all she could do to grab her checkbook and to get away. It happened every time Cindy had to write her name while others were watching.

It was a beautiful spring afternoon; the bay appeared calm and flat as glass—a perfect day for an invigorating row in his boat. Travis felt great as he glided out into the bay. Within a few minutes, he began to feel more and more strain on the oars with each stroke. The boat seemed to be turning against his will and out of his control. His rowing was doing little, if any, good. He had run into a tide rip, like a river rapids coursing just outside of the otherwise calm bay. Travis had heard of small boat tragedies and now he knew how they could happen. He felt a rising panic as his thoughts raced to consider the dangers in the waters swirling around him. He felt weak and his throat was tight. All he could do was row as hard as he was able and hope and pray for the best. Later, after a half an hour of pulling and straining, he pulled back into the bay. Exhausted, he headed straight to the dock. He had spent energy he didn't know he had.

Tom, Cindy, and Travis were each experiencing intense degrees of anxiety. But their respective anxieties meant something different to each of them. Travis knew perfectly well why he was anxious: he was scared of drowning. Tom, on the other hand, had no idea what was happening to him. He feared the worst and felt as if unexpectedly lightning had struck. Cindy, like Travis, knew what was happening. She knew when it would occur but she did not know why it was happening.

Tom and Cindy have a lot in common. They, and millions like them, are suffering from anxiety disorders—raw, uncontrolled anxiety that seems inexplicable, irrational, and interferes with the normal course of their lives. The pattern in which the anxiety manifests itself can be different in each case, but at its core it is nonetheless anxiety. Often, Tom's anxiety seems to appear unexpectedly: while relaxing, sometimes while playing golf, or just before a business meeting. His pattern of anxiety reaction is called *panic disorder*. Cindy knew how she would react to writing in the presence of others. Since it had happened that way a number of times before, she learned to avoid such situations. Cindy suffers from a social phobia called *scriptophobia*. Travis's panic, perhaps experienced at an intensity comparable to that of Tom and Cindy's, is more understandable to us since most of us would feel the same under similar circumstances. Although frightening, the same panic was responsible for having mobilized the intense energy that enabled Travis to pull himself out of the tide rip.

These case examples, and the others that follow, are presented to illustrate that anxiety can be highly debilitating and therefore might be considered abnormal. However, the ability to experience anxiety is quite normal, and, as with Travis, it is even a necessary emotional reaction. Although unpleasant for the most part, this same anxiety response, when experienced within the normal range, can help us accomplish some of our goals. Without the anxiety, Travis could not have sustained the energy and endurance he needed to save himself. On the other hand, under some circumstances, if our fear and anxiety are too intense or too persistent, it will interfere with our ability to perform according to our capabilities. Anxiety can disrupt our ability to concentrate, to remember, and can make us too jittery to perform skilled movements. For many people like Cindy, it leads to active avoidance of any situation that may arouse it further.

In one form or another, anxiety is pervasive in most everyone's lives. Consider just how many of our daily activities are associated with anxiety or are directed toward avoiding or alleviating the feelings of anxiety. A near miss of an accident on the highway, a slip on the stairs, or a reminder of an overdue job not yet completed, each elicits at least a momentary burst of anxiety that alerts us and prepares us to deal with potential emergencies.

We must be able to move freely in our daily activities, to function effectively, and to enjoy the pleasures of life. At the same time, we must maintain the capacity to respond with fear

and anxiety to motivate us when our physical or psychological
well-being is threatened. It is obvious that for normal and effective functioning, some balance must be achieved. However, this
ideal balance of having anxiety present *only* when it is necessary
is not always easy to achieve. For at least some twenty-five million Americans (roughly 10 to 12 percent of the adult population), anxiety has become attached to situations that are not
realistic threats to their well-being as was the case with Cindy.[1]
Or anxiety may seem to come out of nowhere and strike unpre-
dictably as it did with Tom. Each of these conditions, and others,
will be further described in the following pages.

The purpose of this book is to illustrate the various forms of
anxiety and anxiety disorders and to provide some information
and some theory concerning what they are, where they come
from, and how they can be treated when they become a problem. In describing them, I will examine and illustrate the psychological processes by which anxiety becomes attached to situations in such a way that it can significantly interfere with
one's life. Also, I will describe the various treatment procedures
that have been found effective in overcoming many anxiety-
related problems. This book is intended to present the most
current information about anxiety and anxiety disorders. Although anxiety disorders are the most pervasive of psychological disorders, the recent thrust of research and the resultant
accumulation of scientific and clinical knowledge have made
them the most treatable of all psychological conditions today.

ORIGINS OF THE TERMS *ANXIETY, FEAR,* AND *PANIC*

The emotion of anxiety is universally experienced by virtually all humans and by most animals. In all cultures and across
all times, anxiety and fear have been significant factors in the
lives of humans. Although we cannot say for sure that anxiety is
experienced in the same manner by all, it is likely that we, as
members of the human species, share this similar emotional and
physical experience. One way to evaluate similarities across
cultures and down through our history is to examine the words

and their origins, which are used to denote this emotion. For example, our English word *anxiety* is derived from the Latin-based word *angere*, meaning "to choke" or to strangle, a common sensation associated with anxiety. A further derivative and closer to our current broader meaning of anxiety is *anxietas* and *anxius* meaning uneasiness or trouble of mind.[2] As I am sure most readers can attest, these more than two thousand year old terms and their ancient meanings still seem to describe what we experience today as anxiety.

The term *fear*, a variant of this same emotion, has a somewhat different origin. Fear derives from the Germanic or Teutonic languages and comes most directly to English by way of Middle English. Variously written as *faer*, or *feer*, it meant "to lie in wait, to ambush, and to pounce upon." In time, these terms came to mean a reaction to a sudden calamity, or an uneasiness caused by a sense of impending danger.[4] Fear, too, is closely related to the German word *Gefahr*, meaning danger.

These two words—fear and anxiety—have a long history, longer than the roots of our language. In both there is the perception that something harmful is happening, or is about to happen to one; that one is in some form of danger as was Travis.

ANXIETY IN ANCIENT MYTHS

Other terms for this emotional experience derive from ancient myths. Myths are of interest in that they were developed to explain, and to make rational, human experiences and phenomena that were not otherwise explainable. Myths also tell us what were the major life concerns of the people who made them. From the ancient Greeks we have inherited much of the foundation of our Western cultures as well as portions of our language.

The myth surrounding the origin of the term *panic*, for example, comes from the Greek word *panikos*, meaning "of Pan," in reference to the deity Pan. Pan was said to be the guardian of animals, forests, and fields. Among his charges were shepherds while they tended their flocks at night. Pan, being a fun-loving and capricious character, would, just for sport, send waves of terror into the hearts of shepherds in their fields at night. He was also said to frighten wayward travelers in the forest who disturbed his naps.[5] These unexpected cascades of terror appeared to come from unseen sources, and Pan was the likely suspect. Hence the term *panic* for sudden waves of terror that were not associated with imminent danger.

Phobia, another term frequently used throughout this book, is derived from *Phobos*, another Greek deity. Phobos was a son of Aries, the Greek god of war. Greek warriors emblazoned Phobos's visage upon their shields and during battle; they called upon him to help them frighten and rout their enemies.[6]

FEAR OR ANXIETY?

We noted that the terms *fear* and *anxiety* are derived from different languages and relate to somewhat different states. However, it is also the case that they are sometimes used synonymously with each other. Although there is no universally agreed upon technical differentiation between fear and anxiety, general usage and some psychological justification can separate them. In general, anxiety denotes a sense of danger or foreboding and a troubled mind. Something is not right, but the source of the concern is unclear. Something bad "might" happen, but just what and when is unknown.

On the other hand, fear tends to denote a feeling that something bad *is* going to happen, that there is an imminent danger looming. Fear is a response to a more readily identifiable threat that is about to happen. Running from a bear in the woods, for example, represents fear; not leaving home lest a calamity of some sort *might* occur would describe anxiety.

Martin Seligman, a prominent psychological theorist in this area, encompasses some of the above differences into his concept of *predictability*.[7] Seligman believes that the central factor that can differentiate fear from anxiety is the predictability of the source of the threat to which one responds. That is, when an object or situation provides a clear signal or threat or danger and is therefore predictable, the acute emotional state experienced is called *fear*. However, anxiety is seen as "the chronic fear that occurs when a threatening event is in the offing but is unpredictable."[8] Without predictability or clarity of the stimulus, a more chronic and pervasive state of anxiety would exist since the person would be unable to determine exactly what the threat was or when it might occur.

Following this line of differentiation, another characteristic often cited is that if a response is made to a situation that is a "realistic" threat and therefore is seen as rational and functional, it is said to be fear; whereas if a response is made to a stimulus that is not seen as a realistic threat and the response therefore is considered irrational and dysfunctional, it is called anxiety.

Although there are no general definitions that can differentiate between the terms *fear* and *anxiety*, often there are cases when such definitions do not work. For example, when is a snake a realistic and predictable threat and therefore a cause of fear, and when is it unrealistic and unpredictable and therefore a cause of anxiety? A person in the middle of a violent thunderstorm who is concerned about being struck by lightning could be said to be fearful. However, a person who is concerned about being injured when and if a thunderstorm comes sometime in the future might be considered anxious. It is less clear what to call one's apprehension and trembling when going to the dentist. Is it a realistic or an unrealistic response? Is the outcome predictable or unpredictable? Certainly, it can be either, depending upon the condition of one's teeth, the particular dentist, one's past experiences with dentists, and one's sensitivity to pain and discomfort.

FREUD'S CONCEPT OF ANXIETY

Before leaving this discussion of terminology, some variations of these concepts proposed by Sigmund Freud should be noted. It was Freud who, to a large extent, made us aware of the powerful role that anxiety has in affecting our daily lives. He popularized the very term *anxiety* (or *angst*) in the psychological and the popular literature.[9] Anxiety played a central role in Freud's theory of personality in general and psychopathology in particular. He saw anxiety very much as we described it; that is, a "danger signal" alerting the ego of impending threat or harm. Depending upon the locus of the source of threat, Freud proposed three types of anxiety: reality anxiety, neurotic anxiety, and moral anxiety. Anxiety resulting from the perception of threat from the external environment was called *reality anxiety*, or fear as we've defined it. When the source of threat to the ego was internally generated from unconscious impulses and forbidden desires, it was termed *neurotic anxiety*. This differentiation corresponds to our general definition of anxiety in that no apparent or externally identifiable source is evident and is not tied to specific objects. Further, neurotic anxiety could take on different forms or intensities, resulting in phobias or panic reactions. Freud proposed yet a third type of anxiety which resulted from unconscious conflicts between the id impulses and the superego or the "moral" portion of one's personality. This type was referred to as *moral anxiety*, and is generally interpreted as shame or guilt.[10] In this section, I have reviewed several definitions and differentiations of the terms *anxiety* and *fear*. There are yet other usages and definitions, some of which will be introduced in Chapter 2, where origins of fears and anxiety are discussed. For our present purposes, fear will be used to indicate an unpleasant emotional reaction in response to an identifiable external stimulus or situation which is perceived as posing a threat. Anxiety is seen as a similar reaction but where the source of threat is not readily apparent. Although the choice of which term to use is largely an arbitrary preference, it is important to remember that the response, or what the individual experiences, is essentially the same.

WHAT ARE FEAR AND ANXIETY?

Just what are fear and anxiety? How do we know when we are anxious? How do we know when someone else is anxious or fearful? What is it that leads us to conclude that we are anxious?

To begin to answer these questions, we must first realize that fear and anxiety are not things. No one has ever seen a "fear" or an "anxiety," although we all seem to know what they are. To understand more about these states we need to examine what makes them up, as in this typical fear description:

> I had trouble concentrating, keeping my mind on the talk I was about to give. I kept thinking that I was going to forget everything, that I would stutter, freeze, and just stand there blubbering before the class. I knew that I would not be able to answer any questions. My heart was racing, my mouth was dry and my throat was tight, and I felt like I would choke. My hands were so sweaty that they stuck to my notes. My legs felt like rubber and my hands were trembling. I wanted to walk—no, run out of there immediately.

We have all probably felt something like that at some time. This pattern of fear responses is called the *fight-or-flight syndrome*.[11] As part of our biological "survival kit," we are both blessed and plagued with a physiology that rushes to our aid in times of need when a threat or danger is perceived. When we perceive threat, a complex series of bodily changes take place. These changes prepare us to handle the threat: either to fight it or to flee from it. In the long history of our species, those beings who were not equipped to respond with increased energy and strength did not survive long enough to procreate. Those whose bodies reacted in ways that facilitated their ability to fight their attackers or to escape from them survived and became our ancestors. This same capacity has been passed on to us, but it does not discriminate well between threats that truly endanger our lives and those that endanger only our psyches. Unfortunately, the body responds in the same fashion, whatever the source of the perceived threat.

THE COMPONENTS OF FEAR AND ANXIETY

There are three partially independent response systems operating to make our survival system work best for us. These three components involve: (1) the cognitive or thinking processes, (2) the physiological or bodily change processes, and (3) the behavioral component that constitutes our bodily movements. Each of these components interacts with each other component, and, when integrated, provide us with an effective system for handling threats. Let's look separately at each of these systems.

Cognitive Component

First among the systems is the cognitive component. This involves our mental experience, our thoughts about what is happening to us, how we feel, and what we can do, if anything, about the threat.

Examples of the cognitive component of anxiety would include such thoughts as: What was that noise? What is going to happen to me now? What if I mess up and make a fool of myself? I hope I don't trip and fall off the stage! How am I going to get out of here—I'd better run.

When potentially threatening information is perceived, one of the first things to happen is that a *cognitive appraisal* process begins in which one attempts to evaluate the potential consequences of the impending event.[12] Often it is at this point that initial or anticipatory components of anxiety or fear begin. To the extent that the person is either unsure of the outcome or expects it to be negative, the anxiety or fear process is set in motion. This appraisal process can happen instantaneously or it can evolve more slowly as with anticipation of an impending event. This latter, more slowly developing cognitive anxiety, is referred to as *anticipatory anxiety*. For example, when a person makes a dental appointment, perhaps for the first time in several years, a common response is that thoughts may occur concerning what might happen: Will I have cavities? Will the dentist want to fill them? Will it hurt? Will the dentist give me a bad time for not brushing and flossing enough? When thoughts such as these are experienced in anticipation of an event, potential threat is anticipated, our physiology begins to enter the picture, and bodily changes are induced.

Physiological Component

Accompanying anticipatory thoughts about what might occur, and sometimes preceding them, are physiological responses. These responses typically include increases in heart rate, perspiration on our palms and face, muscle tensions, dry mouth, and queasy feelings in our stomachs. These bodily changes are integral parts of the fight-or-flight system and are the result of the activation of one portion our *autonomic nervous system* (ANS). The ANS is that portion of the nervous system responsible for the essentially automatic regulation of many of our internal bodily functions. The ANS is divided into two divisions, which, for the most part, act antagonistically to one another. That is, when one portion is most active, the other is relatively inhibited and vice versa. Overall, these two systems serve to maintain a balance among our internal physical systems and among many other critical functions. Thus, the ANS is intimately involved in fear and anxiety responses.

The *sympathetic nervous system* (SNS) is that branch of the ANS most often involved in fear or anxiety. It is called *sympathetic* because it is the portion that comes to our aid (in sympathy) when we need immediate help with a stressor. It prepares us for meeting emergencies or to physically deal with threats. This preparation helps us to cope with emergencies by mobilizing energy resources and is the source of the fight-or-flight response. When an event is cognitively appraised as being threatening, neural impulses are sent to a center in the adrenal gland which, in turn, release the hormones *epinephrine* (adrenaline) and *norepinephrine* (noradrenaline) into the bloodstream where they are circulated to various organ systems that they stimulate. The physical changes we perceive when we are anxious or frightened are partially a result of these hormones that stimulate organs innervated by the SNS. Table 1 lists the effects of this SNS stimulation. As can be seen, activation of the SNS typically

TABLE 1
Autonomic Nervous System Effects on Bodily Systems[a]

Organ system	Sympathetic branch	Parasympathetic branch
Eyes/pupils	Dilate	Constrict
Heart rate	Increases	Decreases
Bronchia/lungs	Dilate	Constrict
Salivary glands	Reduce saliva (thick)	Increase saliva (watery)
Stomach	Inhibits function	Stimulates function
Adrenal medulla	Secretes epinephrine and norepinephrine	No effect
Sweat glands (in hands and feet)	Increase sweating	No effect
Bloodflow	Increases to skeletal muscles	No effect

[a]The patterns described here are general responses but there are many individual variations in response to stresses or threats.

involves an increase in heart rate, thereby increasing blood circulation; the liver is stimulated to release glycogen as blood sugar to facilitate muscle strength and endurance; bronchioles in the lungs are dilated for more air; and increased sweating occurs and eliminates energy wastes and releases heat.

These ANS effects are broadly dispersed throughout the body, affecting many organ systems and tending to persist for some time. You have most likely noticed, that, when startled or frightened, your heart continues to race even after the danger is gone. This lingering arousal experienced after the threat is due to the fact that the adrenaline continues to circulate in your bloodstream and takes some time to diminish or run itself off.

This sudden emergency rush of energy is thought to have been essential to the survival of our evolutionary ancestors in preparing them to meet many physical dangers. Today, these functions can be extremely useful when we are confronted with a physical danger necessitating strength, endurance, or speed.

However, such reactions are not always helpful, and can interfere with our lives, particularly when we need to use our head rather than our feet.

The *parasympathetic nervous system* (PNS) is the branch of the ANS that is usually reciprocal or oppositional to the SNS. Its function is largely to conserve energy, and it is most active when we are calm, quiet, and relaxed. For example, heart rate is slowed, blood pressure is reduced, and digestion is facilitated (see Table 1). You may have noted that at times when you feel upset or anxious, you do not feel like eating, or if you do eat, the food seems to sit in your stomach undigested. This is because the SNS is most active, and the PNS, whose function is to aid digestion, is slowed down.

Although, for the most part, the PNS does not enter into fear responses, there is a notable exception. In occasional cases of extreme fright or shock, and for some people fearful of blood or injury, a strong PNS response is seen, resulting in lowered blood pressure and dizziness or fainting.[13,14] This unique fainting response will be described in greater detail in Chapter 4.

In this discussion of the components of fear and anxiety, one might get the impression that the cognitive and physiological components act independently. As we will see later, to some extent they do operate separately, but they also interact with one another as parts of a feedback loop. When we perceive some impending threat, we might initiate "anxious thoughts" that serve as perceived threats. In turn, these thoughts, particularly if they persist, can stimulate activation of the ANS and lead to the physical responses just described. On the other hand, we might perceive our heart rate increase which, in turn, can lead to our thinking, "I must be anxious," since in our past experience, when anxious or fearful, we felt a rapid pulse. Thus, as we monitor our thoughts, we may stimulate our physical state, and as we perceive our physical state changing, we may stimulate our cognitive thoughts of anxiety. Furthermore, these perceptions of anxiety often lead us to want to *do* something that instigates the third or behavioral component of fear and anxiety.

Overt Behavioral Component

The third component defining anxiety or fear responses is more public. It involves observable behavior resulting from skeletal muscle responses. These responses include bodily movements, such as physical attempts to avoid or to escape from the threatening situation. Examples of overt *avoidance responses* might include the steps a person who is fearful of snakes would take to avoid the natural habitats of snakes. For example, the person might detour around grassy areas or weed patches in an open field. Similarly, the person fearful of closed spaces might climb 20 flights of stairs to avoid entering an elevator.

In situations where avoidance is not possible, the fearful person might exhibit *escape behavior*, such as running or turning away from the threat. In each of these cases, the escape or avoidance behaviors serve to reduce the person's felt anxiety.

We often find ourselves in threatening situations where escape or avoidance responses are either impossible or are not practical for various reasons. In such situations, we might see other behavioral signs of anxiety or fear, such as trembling hands, shaky or stammering speech, fidgeting and squirming, and a variety of such mannerisms.

Interactions of the Three Components

In many threat situations, whether physical or social, we experience some portion of each of the three response components. When we suddenly come upon a precipitous cliff and look over, we may say to ourselves, "I hope I don't fall." Then we may feel our heart begin to beat rapidly and we physically back away. In cases such as this, there is little question about labeling the overall reaction as fear. However, such consistency among the components is not always evident. A variety of situational constraints can override expression of some of the components, leaving the label of fear in doubt. For example, a person who delivers a speech in front of a class may experience anticipatory anxious thoughts such as, "I hope I don't mess up. Will the class laugh at me? I wish I could leave." These thoughts may be accompanied by physiological responses of increased heart rate, a dry mouth, and sweaty hands. However, if the speaker's class grade is dependent upon giving the speech, and flight is a sure way to look foolish, then the person might give the speech. If the anxiety is not too severe, he may be able to present the appearance of being calm and controlled. To outside observers, this speaker may appear calm since they can neither read his thoughts nor see his heart racing. Nonetheless, the person feels anxious, although privately so. At more intense levels of threat, and for severely phobic individuals, we are likely to see greater consistency among the response systems. However, at lesser levels of intensity, the person might well be able to mask his or her behavioral expression of anxiety and give the appearance of being calm and self-assured. Under these conditions the three systems will not appear to be consistent.

WHAT DETERMINES IF ANXIETY IS NORMAL OR ABNORMAL?

Although the experience of anxiety or fear is a necessary and normal part of life, there are times when it becomes such a problem that it must be considered beyond the range of a normal response. Thus, a frequently posed question concerning anxiety is "How do you know when something as common and pervasive as anxiety is no longer 'normal'?" In other words, when does normal anxiety become abnormal? Unfortunately, there is no easy answer and no formula for determining abnormality. Anxiety is often a normal and a necessary part of life. Indeed, in many situations it is abnormal *not* to experience anxiety. Thus, to call anxiety *abnormal*, one must consider a number of factors. These factors include: the frequency with which it occurs, its chronicity or the duration of occurrence, the rationality of the response, one's ability to control its effects, and its disruption of normal life routines. Each of these factors must be evaluated separately and in combination. Seldom is a single factor likely to give a sufficient picture for this determination. In the following section, we will discuss each of these issues.

Frequency of Occurrence

For the experience of anxiety to be considered abnormal, it must be repetitive. A single or infrequent occurrence of an event is unlikely to be considered a significant problem. For example, a person highly fearful of heights who lives in a flat terrain, in a town with only single-story buildings, is unlikely to experience fear of heights under normal circumstances. A problem would exist only if this person's life circumstances changed such that he or she was required to visit an area with heights. For example, if this person had to move permanently to a city full of skyscrapers, then this fear might be considered abnormal since it would now constitute a problem.

Similarly, many people experience an attack of intense anxiety, sometimes of sufficient intensity to be considered a panic attack.[15] However, for the majority of these people, it is a one-time or an infrequent occurrence; it comes and then goes. Most people do not worry about it for long and the experience is forgotten. Even such an intense attack of panic may not be considered abnormal if it is infrequent.

Chronicity

A second condition to consider is how long an anxiety reaction persists. If a person has a fear reaction to some traumatic event, such as an earthquake, this reaction, of course, would be considered normal, at least initially. However, if others who experienced the same event have recovered, but this person continues to feel anxiety and apprehension over the possibility of another quake's occurring, and if this feeling persists for months, this situation might be considered abnormal and a problem to be concerned about. Similarly, a high proportion of young children develop fears of the dark, of being left alone, and of animals. For children, these are not considered abnormal reactions although they can pose problems for the child. However, the vast majority of these fears are outgrown with time and experience. For those whose childhood fears persist well beyond the expected age range or onward into adulthood, the fear could be considered abnormal.

Rationality

Another issue concerns how rational the anxiety or fear response is; that is, is the response in proportion to the actual threat or danger to the individual? The response of terror at climbing a three-foot ladder would seem irrational. Feeling panic stricken during and immediately following an earthquake would appear expected and rational. Feeling chronic panic over the prospect of another quake three years later would not appear so rational. Of course, it is not easy to gain a consensus on what is rational and what is not. How do we classify a fear of being on a seven-foot ladder or the continued fear two weeks following a quake? These certainly are the gray areas.

Control over Reaction

A hallmark of abnormal anxiety problems is that the reaction exceeds the person's ability to maintain self-control. If the person experiences fear of heights, but is able to control his or her reaction sufficiently to climb a ladder or a flight of stairs when necessary, the experience may be unpleasant but, under normal circumstances, is controllable. Intense anxiety that seems to strike out of nowhere, that seems to take control of the person, or for which the person feels that control is waning, would be considered more toward the direction of abnormal anxiety. This issue of ability to control the anxiety leads to the final criterion of what defines abnormal fear—the extent to which it affects one's daily life.

Life Disruption and Avoidance

The single factor that is perhaps most indicative of whether an anxiety experience is to be considered abnormal and a psychological problem is the extent to which it interferes with and diminishes a person's life functioning. A condition that occurs frequently, that is chronic, that seems not to be a rational response, and over which the person has little or no control, is in all likelihood going to limit that person's life. Each of the anxiety disorders has this feature by definition: it interferes with the normal routine of a person's life. The degree of interference varies for the disorders. For example, some simple phobias may be successfully avoided under usual circumstances with minimal life disruption. A fish phobic may have to avoid pet shops and aquariums, will be unable to go on fishing trips, and may have to avoid some nature programs on TV. However, this may be a minimal disruption for many persons. On the other hand, it is not uncommon for agoraphobics to fear ever leaving the house alone. They cannot attend theaters or gatherings of strangers, they avoid all public conveyances and shopping in grocery or department stores. Clearly, anxiety disrupts and affects the quality of their lives.

Anxiety disorders can diminish significantly a person's quality of life in many ways. Recently, the extent of this diminished quality of life was examined by a team of researchers from the New York State Psychiatric Institute. Jeffrey Markowitz and his colleagues analyzed psychiatric diagnostic interviews of some 18,000 adults representing five communities in the United States.[16] In their analyses, they found that individuals who had received the diagnosis of panic disorder, when compared with persons without panic disorder, reportedly were in poorer health, spent less time on hobbies, were more likely to have marital and alcohol problems, and were more likely to be financially dependent on others. The distress they experienced was also reflected in the fact that they used emergency medical services more than others and fully 20 percent of these panic disordered persons had attempted suicide.[17]

These quality of life problems may also be related to longevity of life. William Coryell and his colleagues found that patients with panic disorder were at greater risk of early death either by suicide or by cardiovascular disorders.[18] Although it is currently impossible to determine if the impaired quality of life and the existence of chronic diseases are the cause or the effect of the anxiety, most researchers today see these two conditions affecting one another. Consequently, illness and chronic disease can contribute to anxiety disorders while, at the same time, chronic and intense anxiety may cause or make existing illnesses worse.

An additional way in which anxiety disorders can erode a person's health and quality of life is through the medical avoidances they cause. Upward of 20 percent of the adult population has, at one time, avoided attending needed dental treatment on account of fear.[19,20] Furthermore, a similar proportion of adults have avoided some aspect of medical care because of fear.[21] Not only is a person's general quality of life diminished, but his or her health may suffer as well owing to unrealistic and unnecessary fears.

> Gertrude was a 68-year-old recently retired teacher. She held a master's degree and had spent her adult working life helping young people with problems. She was totally on top of all areas of her life except one: she had developed a morbid fear of doctors—a phobia. Through a series of unfortunate tragic events, including watching a fellow worker die of a chronic disease, attending her father in the hospital, who eventually died, and abruptly finding that her own physician of 20 years had suddenly died, Gertrude developed a full-blown phobia of medical doctors. When one is well, such a phobia is not a problem. But, when you break your arm, as Gertrude did, it becomes a major problem. For four days, she avoided having the arm examined. Finally, when she could bear the pain no longer, she went to the local clinic, but only when she knew the doctor was gone and only a nurse would be present.

In this case, the phobia was not life threatening, but it could have been had the ailment been another serious condition that relies upon early diagnosis for successful treatment. Not only a person's quality of life can be compromised by such phobias, the life itself can be threatened.

THE ANXIETY DISORDERS: A BRIEF SKETCH

To introduce the various anxiety disorders to be described throughout this book, a brief description of each of the major anxiety conditions follows. This overview will help the reader to follow the commentary when various diagnoses are mentioned prior to their more detailed descriptions, which will be presented in Chapters 4 through 7.

Simple phobia: Phobia is an exaggerated, irrational fear in response to a specific object or situation which is out of proportion to the actual threat or danger. In defining this term, Isaac Marks, a British expert on phobias, notes that phobia is "a special form of fear which: (1) is out of proportion to dangers of the situation, (2) cannot be explained or reasoned away, (3) is beyond voluntary control, and (4) leads to the avoidance of the feared situation."[22]

Social phobia: Like simple phobia, social phobia is an exaggerated, irrational response to a specific situation. In this case, the situation involves other people. The defining characteristic of social phobia is that phobic persons fear that other people will observe them and make a negative evaluation of them or their performance. Cindy's scriptophobia, illustrated at the beginning of this chapter, was a type of social phobia.

Panic disorder: The person with panic disorder experiences periodic paroxysms of panic and terror. Some of these terrors seem to come literally out of nowhere, without warning or cues. Tom's attack of panic while relaxing after a difficult day was a case of panic disorder. Although many persons experience an occasional attack, some experience them with such frequency that they become disruptive to life.

Agoraphobia: Agoraphobia means literally *fear of open spaces.* Although this is somewhat of a misnomer, it does convey the fact that agoraphobics often are unable to venture out of their houses. They come to fear being in public places and/or being out alone. One of the things they fear most is having a panic attack while outside. Many agoraphobics also have panic disorder.

Obsessive-compulsive disorder: Obsessions are persistent and repetitive thoughts that seem to intrude themselves into a person's consciousness. Obsessive thoughts can be so intrusive that some people are unable to think of much else. Compulsions are repetitive acts or rituals that are enacted over and over. If prevented from enacting the ritual, the person becomes exceedingly anxious. Often, obsessive thoughts lead to compulsive behaviors. Obsessions concerning infestation with germs might lead a person to do repetitive hand washing and house cleaning.

Generalized anxiety disorder: The person who is constantly in a state of worry, tension, and anxiety, even when there is no apparent stimulus causing it, is said to be suffering from generalized anxiety disorder. The anxiety is pervasive, it happens everywhere. It is as if the person brings it with him or her and it pervades all aspects of that person's life.

Posttraumatic stress disorder: Although most people subjected to severely traumatic situations, such as natural disasters, war, or physical assault, show an adverse emotional reaction, some people have such extensive reactions that they become debilitated. In some ways, the reaction is like generalized anxiety disorder. However, the person with PTSD may have flashbacks to the trauma, and situations recalling any degree of similarity to the original trauma may cause a total reenactment of the trauma response.

These forms of anxiety constitute the anxiety disorders. They disrupt people's lives, cause no end of misery, and endanger health. They may drive people to abuse alcohol and other drugs out of attempts to find relief, and for some, they may even lead to suicide. In the following chapters, I will describe these conditions, where they come from, and what can be done about them.

SUMMARY AND CONCLUSIONS

Anxiety and fear are part of our evolutionary legacy. Although they are always unpleasant, both are necessary for our very survival. Our ancestors observed that when faced with danger, they experienced choking and constricting sensations. From these sensations is derived our current term of anxiety. Anxiety and panic must have been prominent throughout history. To the Greeks and others, such powerful effects as experienced in panic could only be instigated by supernatural forces. These potent experiences must have been acts of the gods, Pan and Phobos.

Fear and anxiety pervade our lives as much as ever and are experienced as three related components: the cognitive or mental experience, the physiological activity in our autonomic nervous systems, and the avoidance and escape-related behaviors. When the activation of these anxiety response systems becomes so intense or pervasive as to significantly disrupt a person's normal daily functioning, they can be considered abnormal and as such can be diagnosed into one of the seven anxiety disorders.

Anxiety is irrevocably a major part of human experience and human nature. As such we should examine its roots, how it develops and attaches to us and to objects that we associate with, and how it sometimes appears to flare up out of nowhere. In the next chapter, I will examine the roots of anxiety.

REFERENCES

1. American Psychiatric Association, "Phobias" (Washington, D.C.: American Psychiatric Press, 198).
2. *Oxford English Dictionary,* s.v. "anxiety."

3. Ibid., *anxietas*.

4. Ibid., s.v. "fear."

5. David Barlow, *Anxiety and Its Disorders* (New York: Guilford Press, 1988).

6. Paul Errera, "Some Historical Aspects of the Concept, Phobia," *Psychiatric Quarterly* 36 (1962): 325–336.

7. Martin Seligman, *Helplessness: On Depression, Development, and Death* (New York: W. H. Freeman, 1975).

8. Ibid., p. 112.

9. Ernst Jones, *The Life and Works of Sigmund Freud* (Garden City, N.Y.: Doubleday, 1961).

10. Richard Price, *Abnormal Behavior: Perspectives in Conflict*, 2nd ed. (New York: Holt, Rinehart & Winston, 1978).

11. Walter Cannon, *Bodily Changes in Pain, Hunger, Fear and Rage*, 2nd ed. (New York: Appleton-Century-Crofts, 1929).

12. Richard Lazarus, *Psychological Stress and the Coping Process* (New York: McGraw-Hill, 1966).

13. Ronald Kleinknecht and Joseph Lenz, "Blood/Injury Fear, Fainting, and Avoidance of Medical Treatment: A Family Correspondence Study," *Behaviour Research and Therapy* 27 (1989): 537–547.

14. Lars-Goran Öst, Ulf Sterner, and Inga-Lena Lindahl, "Physiological Responses in Blood Phobics." *Behaviour Research and Therapy* 22 (1984): 109–117.

15. G. Ron Norton, J. Dorward, and B. Cox, "Factors Associated with Panic in Non-clinical Subjects," *Behavior Therapy* 17 (1986): 239–252.

16. Jeffrey Markowitz, Myrna Weissman, Robert Ouellette, Jennifer Lish, and Gerald Klerman, "Quality of Life in Panic Disorder," *Archives of General Psychiatry* 46 (1989): 984–992.

17. Myrna Weissman, Gerald Klerman, Jeffrey Markowitz, and Robert Ouellette, "Suicidal Ideation and Suicidal Attempts in Panic Disorder and Attacks," *New England Journal of Medicine* 321 (1989): 1209–1214.

18. William Coryell, Robert Noyes, and J. Clancy, "Excessive Mortality in Panic Disorder: Comparison with Primary Unipolar Depression," *Archives of General Psychiatry* 43 (1982): 701–703.

19. Peter Milgrom, Louis Fiset, Sandra Melnick, and Philip Weinstein, "The Prevalence and Practice Management Consequences of Dental Fear in a Major U.S. City," *Journal of the American Dental Association* 116 (1988).

20. Peter Milgrom, Philip Weinstein, Ronald Kleinknecht, and Tracy Getz, *Treating Fearful Dental Patients: A Patient Management Handbook* (Reston, Va.: Reston Press, 1988).

21. Ronald Kleinknecht and Joseph Lenz, "Blood/Injury Fear, Fainting, and Avoidance of Medical Treatment: A Family Correspondence Study," *Behaviour Research and Therapy* 27 (1989): 537–547.

22. Isaac Marks, *Fears and Phobias* (New York: Academic Press, 1969).

CHAPTER 2

The Roots of Anxiety

The roots of any emotion that pervades so many aspects of our lives and that serves us in so many ways must be highly complex. Indeed, the roots of anxiety are wide and deep, tapping into our long evolutionary history while also branching into the more recent history of uniquely human mental processes. To understand the why and the wherefore of anxiety, we will need to examine information ranging from our genetics to our environmental experiences. The raw materials from which we, as humans, develop are biological units and, consequently, we are similar to lower animals in many ways. Accordingly, we can look to knowledge derived from animal experiments to more fully understand some of our own biological and psychological processes. However, as humans we have evolved beyond strict reliance on instinctive biological processes for our survival and general functioning. Our greater brain power and its resultant higher mental processes render us more capable of, and also dependent on, learning to adapt to changing environments. Furthermore, we can create environments, not just react to them. We can also plan, think ahead, and anticipate the future. However, with these same abilities to think of the future, we can anticipate problems that "might" happen. This anticipation helps to protect us but allows us to worry, whether we need to or not. This ability to anticipate and to project into the future can be the source of many anxiety problems.

In our exploration of the roots of anxiety, we will begin examining data derived from animals, some of which might have implications for understanding ourselves. Then we will review some human research findings that involve learning and thinking processes as they figure in anxiety development.

Fear and anxiety, like many other traits of human behavior, can develop from several sources. These sources may act individually in some cases or they may act in combination to result in a specific fear or anxiety state. Thus, some conditions may be caused primarily by physiological processes whereas psychological processes may predominate in others. In this section I will discuss the various sources individually and then present a theoretical position that attempts to integrate some of the sources.

BIOLOGICAL ORIGINS: ANIMAL DATA

It is my belief that understanding animal behavior patterns that appear similar to those seen in humans will help us to understand many of the basic behavioral processes that are associated with fear and anxiety. We should be aware, however, of the fact that human behavior is considerably more complex, and that it may show only remote vestiges of the biologically related behavior patterns seen in lower animals.

"Wired-In" Fear Behavior Patterns

In many species of animals, an innate disposition causes the animal to respond automatically to certain stimuli or stimulus patterns with fearlike behaviors. It is as though a "wired-in" automatic response existed that is activated when certain conditions or stimulus configurations are encountered. Typically, these fear response patterns involve some form of escape or avoidance response and appear to have clear adaptive or survival value for the animal. The animal that does not run or hide from its predators will not survive and, of course, will not be able to reproduce its species.

The Hawk-Effect

One such purported phenomenon is termed the *Hawk-effect*. Two prominent European ethologists, Niko Tinbergen and Konrad Lorenz, observed that young ducks and geese responded with fear when they saw a hawklike image soaring overhead. The hawk, of course, would be a natural predator of small ducks and geese. The researchers also observed that if the hawklike image were reversed so that its long tail portion became the leading image followed by the shorter end, the young birds did not react with fear. This reversed image appeared more like that of a flying goose, which would not pose a predatory threat. These ethologists suggested that there is an innate fear mechanism in the brains of young birds that is activated when certain visual patterns are perceived that are associated with danger.

Further investigation of the hawk effect has qualified this conclusion, since it has been determined that the fear response is probably not elicited by the hawk image *per se*. Rather, it appears to be the result of the pattern of a rapid increase in visual stimulation which would be more likely to result from a hawklike image approaching with its short neck and wide wings followed by its narrow tail. The reverse image would show more gradual stimulation.[1] Other non-hawklike images that swooped toward young chicks and that also resulted in a rapid increase of visual stimuli have been found to elicit the fear or escape responses as well.

Fear of Facial Threats

A threatening face is another stimulus pattern shown to elicit fear and avoidance behaviors. In a classic study, Gene Sackett investigated innate fear responses in young rhesus monkeys.[2] These monkeys were reared in total social isolation from other monkeys or humans. By isolating them, Sackett eliminated the possibility that they might learn to fear faces of other monkeys. His method involved projecting into the monkeys' cages pictures of a number of stimuli and observing the animals' responses. The results indicated that the pictures showing another monkey presenting a threatening posture and facial expression produced more disturbed, fearful, or withdrawn behavior in the young monkeys than other pictures showing infants playing, fearful monkeys, geometric patterns, or living rooms.

More important for demonstrating the innateness of the fear response to the threatening pictures was the clear maturational or developmental effect. Up to two months of age, the infant monkeys showed no fear or disturbance to the threatening pictures. In fact, they appeared to enjoy the threatening pictures and would press a lever in order to view them. However, by 2 to 2.5 months, the same threat pictures began to elicit fear and disturbed behavior. This fear behavior peaked at about 3 months and declined rapidly during the 4th month. During the 2.5- to 3-month period, the animals also drastically reduced their lever pressing to view these threat slides. But by 4 months of age, the lever pressing again increased, suggesting that they no longer had such fear reactions. This study suggests that there may be certain stimulus configurations that innately represent threats that produce automatic, reflexive fear reactions. These innate fear reactions would be particularly adaptive in the young animals who may not yet be physically mature enough or have not yet learned to protect themselves by other means.

Scared Stiff

The widely observed fear-related phenomenon called *tonic immobility* (TI) provides yet another way of looking at the biological basis of fear behavior in animals. Tonic immobility, also called *animal hypnosis* and *death feigning*, results when an animal is physically restrained or held down. After about 15 seconds of initial struggle, the animal becomes motionless. When released, the animal will remain rigid except for muscle tremors in the legs and will appear to be asleep or "hypnotized." Once TI is induced, it will last anywhere from several minutes to several hours. The duration of the response varies by species and can be altered by a number of experimental procedures. This phenomenon is believed to be a kind of fear response since many stimuli that produce fear also increase the duration of TI. For example, presenting loud noises to the animal or injecting it with adrenaline will result in an increase in the length of time the animal remains immobile.[3]

Since TI has been found in a large portion of the animal kingdom, from insects to reptiles to primates, researchers suggest that the response has evolved as an innate defense against predators. Once captured by a predator, if the animal, after its initial struggle, becomes motionless, the predator often will lose interest and become distractable, allowing the prey to escape. Although it is a rather large inferential leap and there are no definitive data to support the contention, some investigators have suggested that when human beings are "scared stiff" or paralyzed with fear they evidence a human equivalent of TI that is seen in lower animals.

Genetic Transmission of Fear

The previous section provided data suggesting that fear reactivity, at least among lower animals, may have a biologically adaptive function that serves to maintain the species. The various forms of fear response described were seen as generally characteristic of a given species, although responses similar to TI are seen in a wide variety of species. Also, there are within species differences in fear reactivity. For example, some dogs appear shy and reactive whereas others appear quite fearless. Using a genetic approach to investigate these differences, a number of researchers have instituted *crossbreeding* in attempts to produce fear variations within a given species. The general procedure is first to identify several animals, some of which appear to be naturally fearful or timid and others which appear fearless. Some of the fear-related characteristics often sought in these animals are reactivity to new or novel environments, persons, or noises. The "fear" responses seen include huddling, cringing, or the tendency to withdraw when placed in a new situation. Once the fearful and nonfearful animals are selected, they are bred with others who also have the same characteristics. If these fear characteristics are genetically transmitted, succeeding generations of fearful animals should become more similar to each other, and more divergent from their opposites— the fearless or nonreactive animals. Successive generations of two strains should become more and more dissimilar with respect to fearlike reactions.

A number of studies, using different species, have shown quite convincingly that through selective breeding, fearful and fearless (reactive and nonreactive) strains can be developed. Crossbreeding experiments have been conducted with a wide variety of animals. Pointer dogs, for example, were bred to be highly responsive to loud noises and to avoid men.[4] Chickens have been selectively bred for the duration that they stay in tonic immobility, suggesting that this fear-related response also has some genetic basis.[5]

With this brief review of some of the biological contributions to fear responsiveness, it is clear that among lower animals fear behavior has strong biological underpinnings. The reactiveness noted here may be similar to trait anxiety seen in humans. Next, we will examine some research concerning the biological or genetic relationships of fear in human behavior.

BIOLOGICAL ORIGINS: HUMAN DATA

Like the lower animals, humans also show wide variations in the propensity to exhibit specific fears and to react to situations with anxiety. In this section, we will examine information suggesting that at least some of this variation stems from a person's biological or genetic makeup. Thus, some people may be born with the predisposition to react to many situations with fear or anxiety.

It is considerably more difficult with humans to isolate the biological influences from the psychological or learning influences. Obviously we cannot rear humans in total isolation from others as Sackett did with his monkeys. Nor can we select persons with and without certain fear-related characteristics and crossbreed them to investigate the hereditary contribution of these response traits. Consequently, we are limited in human research to studying the anxiety problems where and when we find them and with this form of study we are less able to form definitive conclusions.

Furthermore, since humans have few natural predators, we might not expect hereditary components to be as specific as they might be in lower animals. Rather, from an evolutionary point of view, we might expect to observe only remnants or vestiges of specific fears, such as fear of snakes.

Instead of possessing a number of biologically determined specific fears, we see in humans more of a general disposition to react to a variety of situations with fear or anxiety: something more akin to trait anxiety. Such general dispositions to respond with fearlike behavior or anxiety are identifiable in humans from very early ages. When referring to such dispositions with the implication that they are inborn personality patterns the term *temperament* is often used.

Parents, nurses, and pediatricians can all testify that children display distinctly different reaction patterns from the time of birth. To investigate these apparent temperament patterns, a group of researchers intensely studied 141 children over a number of years. Through periodic observation of the children and interviews with the parents, they were able to identify several distinct personality or temperament characteristics that are evident from the first two to three months of life. The patterns appeared to emerge independently of the parents' child-rearing practices and thus appeared to be inborn behavioral patterns.[6]

Among the nine reaction patterns observed, one is particularly relevant to our study of fear and anxiety, because it involves children's responses to new objects or persons presented to them. Some children would respond to strangers or to most any change by withdrawing and displaying fear or worrylike behaviors. Others would show the opposite pattern of accepting changes, approaching new situations and being highly verbal and social with strangers.

Over the years, these patterns remained relatively stable for many of the children. A 6-month old child who, for example, would cry in reaction to a stranger's face, was also likely to be shy and withdrawn at school several years later. These early identified reaction patterns tended to persist over the years, suggesting that these fearlike behavior patterns were inborn temperaments. However, even if inborn, these patterns are potentially modifiable by interactions with parents and others.

More recently, similar observations have been made in different contexts that also suggest that extreme shyness may be an inborn trait. Jerome Kagan, a prominent child psychologist at Harvard, also investigated a group of children over a period of years.[7] He observed that children identified as shy and who tended to withdraw from unfamiliar events at twenty-one months of age also behaved this way in the ensuing years into adolescence and beyond. In his studies, Kagan found that many of these extremely timid children had high and stable heart-rate responses when confronted with new persons or situations. He further noted that approximately one third of the children who were very shy as infants overcame their timidity with age. However, those who changed were not the ones who demonstrated the characteristically high heart rate in response to new situations. In extensions of these studies, Kagan and his colleagues found that when these same shy, inhibited children, who remained that way in later years, were confronted with even mild stresses, they showed greater secretion of norepinephrine and cortisol, two biochemical signs that they were more anxious compared with their opposites—the uninhibited children.[8] These findings suggest that some children are shy from birth, remain that way, and that this shyness is reflected in their withdrawal and inhibited behavior as well as in their secretions associated with activation of the sympathetic portion of the autonomic nervous system. Furthermore, Kagan observed that for most of the children who were highly reactive and inhibited during the first few years of life, chronic environmental stressors were necessary to firmly establish this pattern of behavior as a long-term part of their personalities.

These studies suggest then that there may be inborn patterns of general fearfulness of new or unfamiliar objects or situations and that these traits may persist into later life, especially if the child is subjected to continuing stresses.

Although these intensive, long-term studies of children seem to suggest that some people are born with a tendency to react to the world in shy and fearful ways, it is not possible, from these studies alone, to identify conclusively the cause of these temperament patterns. We do not know if they are the result of particular genetic inheritances, from observational learning, or from such prenatal influences as nutritional or hormonal variations. To look more precisely at possible causal factors, we need to look at the results of twin studies.

Twin studies are particularly useful for exploring genetic-related behaviors. The typical behavioral genetic twin-study procedure is to compare vis-à-vis some behavioral or personality trait the similarities between identical or *monozygotic* (MZ) twins, who share the same genes and are essentially genetic copies of each other. The degree of similarity is usually expressed as a correlation coefficient. A correlation coefficient is a numerical figure that ranges from 0 to 1.0. The greater the similarity between the two twins on the trait in question, the closer the correlation is to 1.0. The same procedure would be done for a group of fraternal or *dizygotic* (DZ) twins who, although born at the same time, are genetically no more similar than regular siblings. If there is a greater degree of similarity between the MZ twin pairs on the trait than between the DZ twins, the difference, if large enough, is taken as evidence that the characteristic is at least partially a result of genetic factors.

In Great Britain, Lader and Wing used the twin-study method to investigate the hereditary influence on patterns of ANS reaction to certain stimuli.[9] As we saw in the first chapter, the ANS (particularly, the sympathetic portion) is the physiological response system most active during fear or anxiety. Lader and Wing exposed two groups of twins (11 MZ and 11 same-sex DZ pairs) to a series of tones and measured several kinds of ANS reactions to these tones. One measure was the degree to which the galvanic skin response (GSR, a measure of sweating and electrical changes in the skin) decreased or habituated over successive presentation of the tones. On the GSR, they found that the correlation of habituation scores between the MZ twins was quite high (.75), whereas the correlation between DZ twins was considerably lower (.13). These results indicate that the ANS of MZ twin pairs tends to react quite similarly. For example, as one twin's response would decrease over time, there was a strong tendency for the co-twin to show a similar decrease in GSR. In contrast, the similarity between the DZ twin pairs was substantially lower. One twin's response would not necessarily be related to how the other twin reacted.

A similar finding was reported for heart-rate response. Again, MZ twins showed high similarity with a correlation of .78, whereas the DZ twins showed a dissimilar reaction. The correlation for the DZ was −.38. The negative sign here indicates that, to some degree, as one twin showed an increase in heart rate, the other might show a decrease; they reacted oppositely.

Since there was the relatively high degree of similarity in physiological response between MZ co-twins who have essentially identical genetic makeup, and the considerably lesser degree of similarity between DZ twins, these results strongly suggest that ANS reactivity is at least partially a function of genetic endowment.

The degree of social introversion or shyness has also been shown to indicate a hereditary relationship. Table 2 shows the results of three twin studies of children, adolescents, and adults. The 1962 study by Shields is of particular interest since he analyzed separately the relationships between those twins who were reared together and those who were raised in different households. Similarities between these pairs would be less likely to be a result of common learning experiences, leaving mainly genetic influences to account for similarities. The correla-

TABLE 2

Correlations Between Twins on Social Anxiety Proneness

Gottesman (1962) Social introversion personality scale[10]	Scarr and Salapatek Home observation of children's shyness[11]	Shields (1962) Introversion inventory[12]
MZ .55	.88	.61[a] .42[b]
DZ .08	.28	−.17

[a]Twins raised separately.
[b]Twins raised together.

tion coefficient for extroversion for those who were raised separately was .61. The MZ group that was raised together showed some but less similarity (.42). The DZ twins who were reared together had a low, negative correlation of −.17, indicating that, to a small degree, they were actually dissimilar or opposite in social extroversion.

These twin studies imply that some facets of anxiety, particularly those relative to social situations, may be due in part to genetic factors. Even though the twin studies did not examine individuals with anxiety disorders *per se*, other studies have. In one such study, Slater and Shields found that within a group of MZ twins, one of whom was diagnosed as suffering from anxiety neurosis or anxiety state, 41 percent of the co-twins also received that same diagnosis. Among the DZ twins, again when one was diagnosed as having anxiety neurosis, only 4 percent of the co-twins received the same diagnosis. When the authors broadened their diagnosis to include more general anxiety traits, which may not have been as severe as the anxiety neurosis, the percentages of similarity increased to 65 percent for the MZ group and to 13 percent for the DZ group.

Recently, twin studies were conducted in Norway by the psychologist Sven Torgersen of Oslo University.[13] Studying 32 pairs of MZ and 53 pairs of DZ twins, he found that in cases in which one MZ twin was diagnosed as suffering from an anxiety disorder, 34 percent of the co-twins also had an anxiety disorder diagnosis. This figure contrasts with only 17 percent of the DZ twins who had shared anxiety disorder diagnoses. However, it is interesting that in the 32 MZ twin pairs in whom both were diagnosed as having anxiety disorders, in no cases did both have the same type of anxiety disorder. That is, if one had panic disorder, the other had something like obsessive-compulsive disorder. Also, it was found that the seeming genetic relationship held for all anxiety disorders studied here except generalized anxiety disorder. (Simple phobia was not included in the study because it has seldom been found to show geneticlike relationships.) This study suggests that anxiety of sufficient severity to cause disorders and disruptions in a person's daily life may have a genetic basis but that the specific type of anxiety problem may be determined by other factors, presumably that person's learning and developmental experiences.

Interesting, too, is the fact that although the same phobias are often found among family members, there is little evidence to suggest a genetic relationship in specific fears or phobias. Torgersen has shown that there is some genetic relationship in reports of common fears.[14] To the extent that genetics are related to the presence of fears and anxieties, the influence appears to be more of a propensity to be highly reactive to unfamiliar or stressful situations and/or to react with anxiety to a wide variety of situations rather than the inheritance of specific disorders and fears. Many researchers of anxiety disorder agree now that what is inherited is a broad vulnerability to overreact to stressors, with specific disorders being shaped by the environment.[15] To explain the development of specific fears and phobias, we now turn to the contribution of our environmental learning experiences.

LEARNING AND CONDITIONING ORIGINS

Although our biological makeup may well have an impact on our capacity to experience fear and anxiety and our tendencies to react to potentially threatening situations with anxiety or fear, it is largely our environmental experiences that determine what we are fearful of and when our anxieties are manifest. In this section, I will present the processes and theoretical explanations that are proposed to describe how these experiences lead to fearful or anxious behavior. Among these processes are included classical conditioning, vicarious or indirect learning, cognitive or thinking processes, and psychodynamic formulations.

Classical Conditioning

The processes of classical conditioning have long been held to be one of the major mechanisms by which anxieties, fears, and phobias are developed. The delineation of conditioning procedures came from the pioneering experiments in which the Russian Nobel Laureate Ivan Pavlov conditioned dogs to salivate to the sound of a metronome or bell (among other stimuli). The basic processes of conditioning involve simultaneously exposing the subject to two different stimuli. One stimulus must be of the nature that it automatically elicits a specific reflexive response. This reflexive response is called the *unconditioned response* (UCR). The stimulus that causes the automatic UCR is called the *unconditioned stimulus* (UCS). The second stimulus, the one paired with the UCS, is such that it initially has no effect on the response in question; that is, by itself it is neutral with respect to the response. This second stimulus is called the *conditioned stimulus* (CS). After several pairings of the CS followed by the UCS, the CS alone acquires the capability of eliciting the response previously caused by the UCS. When the response is elicited by the CS alone, it is called a *conditioned response* (CR).

When applied to fear or emotional conditioning, the UCS can be any stimulus that can cause an automatic emotional reaction in a person. In laboratory experiments, for example, common UCSs include electric shock or frighteningly loud noises. When these stimuli (UCSs) are paired with other nonemotion-arousing stimuli (CSs), the CS alone elicits an emotional anxiety or fear response (CR) in the exposed person.

One of the first and most influential proponents of the conditioning theory of fear and anxiety acquisitions was John B. Watson. Watson's impact on the conditioning view stemmed largely from an experiment in which he and his assistant, Rosalie Raynor, conditioned a young child to fear furry objects and animals.[16] The subject of this experiment was an 11-month-old child named Albert B., often referred to as "Little Albert." At the time of the study in 1920, Albert lived in a foundling home where his mother worked.

As in any conditioning study, the first step was to demonstrate that the subject had no prior fear response to the objects to which he was to be conditioned. Consequently, Watson showed Albert a white rat, a rabbit, a dog, a monkey, masks, and a ball of white cotton. None of these caused any fear reaction in Albert and they were therefore considered neutral with respect to fear.

The conditioning procedure that followed consisted of allowing Albert to play with a white rat that was to be the CS. As Albert reached for the rat, a steel bar was struck with a hammer just behind Albert's head. The loud sound had previously been shown to cause Albert to cry with fear and was therefore the UCS that caused an emotional response. After six presentations of the rat (CS), followed by the gong (UCS), the rat was presented alone as a test trial. At the sight of the rat, Albert began to cry and crawl away. Five days later, the investigators again showed Albert the rat without the gong and again it elicited the crying and withdrawal. From this demonstration, Watson concluded that the rat had become a conditioned stimulus for the elicitation of fear in Albert.

Watson and Raynor then went on to demonstrate *stimulus generalization*. Albert was shown a white rabbit, a dog, a fur coat, cotton, and a Santa Claus mask, none of which at this point had been paired with the UCS. Recall that none of these stimuli had previously caused fear. Now, each furry item that was similar to the rat elicited some fear in Albert. This demonstration of fear conditioning was taken by Watson and other psychologists as proof that fear and anxiety reactions were essentially directly acquired conditioned responses or were acquired by stimulus generalization.

From this demonstration by Watson, coupled with Pavlov's experiments demonstrating the nature and extent of our capacity to acquire CRs to a wide variety of environmental stimuli, the conditioning theory of fear acquisition became established. These early studies were further bolstered by virtually thousands of subsequent fear conditioning studies that clearly showed that fear and anxiety reactions could be conditioned to previously neutral stimuli.

Despite the many laboratory experiments and demonstrations of classically conditioned fear responses, a number of problems became apparent that tempered the earlier enthusiasm in applying this theory to the acquisition of all human fears. Stanley Rachman, of the University of British Columbia, has outlined several arguments against the unqualified acceptance of such conditioning as the only method of fear acquisition.[17,18] Rachman noted that there are numerous well-documented cases in which one would expect fear conditioning to occur but in which it did not. For example, he cited evidence from the World War II bombings of London. Here, the Londoners were presented with numerous traumas and frightening experiences, yet very few developed the conditioned fear reactions that would be expected from the conditioning theory.

Similarly, there are numerous instances in which people have received painful and fear-producing stimulation but fear is not conditioned to the perpetrator nor to other stimuli prominent in the situation. For example, many people have experienced trauma at the dentist's office and from painful medical procedures. Yet only a portion of them develop a fear of these persons or situations.[19]

A further problem with the unqualified acceptance of the conditioning theory is that attempts to replicate Watson's conditioning of Little Albert have not always been successful. Bregman was unable to condition fear in a group of young children to such objects as curtains or geometrically shaped blocks.[20] Similarly, Valentine was unable to elicit conditioned responses to a pair of opera glasses. However, he did obtain signs of fear after pairing a loud whistle with a furry caterpillar.[21] In yet another attempt, English was able to condition fear to a stuffed black cat but not to a wooden duck.[22] These demonstrations suggest that, at least in children, conditioned fear reactions can be obtained to some objects (e.g., furry creatures) but only with difficulty, if at all, to others.

A further point of evidence that serves to limit the general fear conditioning theory is the observation that the distribution of fear in the population is far from what we might expect. For example, fear of snakes was shown to be the most prevalent of common fears. Yet very few people have been directly traumatized by them. On the other hand, fear of dentists is only half as prevalent as fear of snakes. Many people have received direct painful and noxious stimuli during dental treatment, but all do not develop conditioned fear reactions.[23]

A final criticism of the general conditioning theory of fear acquisition comes from the reports of persons who experience fears and phobias. In studies investigating the origins of fears, many fearful subjects were unable to recall any conditioning experiences. Other investigators found that as many as 65 percent of patients who were seeking treatment for phobias reported a conditioning experience associated with the origin of the phobia. For example, Joseph Wolpe found that 65 percent of his patients reported phobia conditioning, whereas Lars-Goran Öst in Sweden found 57.5 percent of his phobic patients reporting such experiences.[24,25] Note that those studies that investigated clinical-level phobias (those for which patients were seeking treatment) showed a preponderance of their subjects attributing their fears to conditioning. On the other hand, those investigators who studied persons with subclinical fears, typically college students, found that their subjects showed lesser percentages of their fears to be based on conditioning experiences and more from vicarious or observational experiences, such as observing others' receiving painful treatment and the like. The suggestion has been put forth that direct conditioning experiences cause the more severe phobic conditions, whereas more common fears result from other vicarious or observational experiences.

The foregoing points of criticism do not disprove that conditioning may be one way in which fears and phobias are acquired. Indeed, there are ample demonstrations, both clinical and experimental, that some fears and phobias develop via conditioning. However, the numerous exceptions limit the theory's generality and all-inclusiveness. Consequently, we must look to other possible sources of fear development.

Vicarious and Informational Sources

Many people report fears of objects and situations that they have never personally encountered, let alone been directly traumatized by. Consequently, the conditioning theory of fear acquisition cannot account for the full range of fears. A second process or series of processes by which fears and anxieties are acquired is that of observational or vicarious learning and direct instruction. That is, rather than experiencing a trauma or being frightened in the presence of a specific stimulus situation, a person can acquire specific fears and phobias by observing another person undergoing the trauma of being harmed or frightened. Just as children learn to imitate the mannerisms and other characteristics of their parents, they can also acquire the emotional reactions they see in others.

There are several studies that show a significant correlation between parents' fears and children's fears. Since through twin studies it does not appear that specific fears are genetically transmitted, these parent–child similarities most likely result from the imitation process.[26] This is exactly what a number of fearful persons report. For example, Jim, a severely needle-phobic person I once treated, ascribed the beginnings of his intense fear reaction to just such a vicarious experience. He recalled that as a 10-year-old child, he and his classmates at school were lined up in the gymnasium where they were all to receive vaccinations. As Jim's turn approached, he recalled an increasing apprehension. The specific experience that cemented his phobic reaction came as the child in front of him was receiving the injection in his arm. Apparently the child jerked away from the nurse and broke off the needle from the syringe. Jim still recalled that child screaming and the needle dangling from his arm. Needless to say, Jim did not wait for his turn nor did he ever go near a needle again for years. This intense fear of needles also led to his total avoidance of dentistry for the next eleven years until he received treatment for the phobia.

Just as Jim had never been hurt or directly frightened by a dentist, many people develop their fears through a variety of indirect processes including stories and even direct instruction, which often includes large doses of exaggeration and misinformation. Direct instruction has long been one means of imparting information to children. Children are enjoined to stay out of the street, to avoid strangers, and not to play with fire. These, of course, are natural hazards to children who must at the very least learn respect for them, if not fear them. However, the line between respect and excessive fear is not always clear to children. Such well-intended instruction can lead in many cases to misinformation that can result in unnecessary fear. Such a process was illustrated in the report of a spider phobic's description of where his fear originated:

> I was given instruction by my mother as to the grave danger involved in the possibility of being bitten by some types of spider. In our yard she took all six children out and told us to stand back and beware. Then she looked in the ivy and carefully caught a black widow. She held it in a container telling how otherwise she would be bitten and die. . . . I saw my first tarantula at a zoo and was told it was capable of killing with one bite.

The transmission of fears through vicarious and informational sources appears to be one of the major means of fear acquisition. However, this theory, too, presents many of the same vulnerabilities noted with the direct conditioning theory. Many persons exposed to such information do not develop fears. Furthermore, very few laboratory-based experimental studies have examined the processes of transmission of significant fears or phobias through these processes. However, ample evidence exists that fears can be eliminated by such vicarious processes as observing a fearless person exposed to the feared object or situation. This process of communicating to the observer that no danger is present appears to involve the same processes as fear development, only the information is reversed.

Taken together, the direct conditioning processes and indirect information or vicarious communication of fears appear to account for most of the cases of fears or phobias. However, some anomalies still remain to be accounted for in these theories. Why, for example, were fears able to be conditioned to furry objects but not to common blocks or geometric shapes? In an attempt to account for some of these questions, a revision of the conditioning theory is proposed in the next section.

Biology and Conditioning: Prepared Fears

In the previous sections, we noted that a biological component may somehow predispose persons to be fearful. We saw that some fears could be acquired by classical conditioning. However, neither of these positions by itself can adequately explain all the observed data concerning the prevalence and characteristics of fears. Martin Seligman of the University of Pennsylvania has attempted to integrate these two positions and thereby account more fully for the differential prevalence of some fears.[27] Seligman's proposal is that humans may be biologically prepared to develop certain specific fears and less prepared to develop others. He contends that certain stimuli, particularly small animals that were dangerous to our evolutionary ancestors, through natural selection have become highly conditionable CSs. Thus, we may be biologically prepared to develop conditioned fear responses to stimuli that in our evolutionary past portended danger. The ability to develop fear readily to these stimuli would help us to avoid them and therefore survive. Snakes and spiders, in particular, are suggested as prepared fear stimuli.[28]

This preparedness theory of fear or phobia acquisition has been used to explain the disproportionately high prevalence of certain fears, such as of snakes, spiders, and other small animals. On the other side, we see relatively fewer specific fears of more posttechnological stimuli even though they are realistically a greater danger. For example, fear of hammers is rare. Yet, many of us have received severe or painful stimulation to our thumbs from hammers. Similarly, as previously noted, fear of dentistry is only half as prevalent as fear of snakes, even though the likelihood of receiving painful stimulation from dentistry is considerably greater than being hurt by or even seeing a snake.

This preparedness theory of fears and phobias as proposed by Seligman further hypothesizes that (1) prepared fears are easily acquired with as little as a single conditioning experience, (2) once developed, they will be quite resistant to extinction, and (3) that prepared conditioned fears will not be diminished by verbally conveyed information—for example, that spiders are not very likely to be harmful.

A number of experimental studies have evaluated this theory. In Sweden, Arne Öhman and Kenneth Hugdahl at the University of Uppsala conducted several conditioning studies comparing the speed of conditioning and the resistance to extinction, once the UCS was no longer paired with the CS. These studies showed that subjects did develop conditioned responses more rapidly to slides of "prepared" stimuli (snakes and spiders) than they did to flowers and other nondangerous objects. However, the conditioned fear reactions to prepared stimuli did not differ from those developed to other, post-technologically dangerous objects such as guns or sparking electric wires. However, in partial support of the theory was the finding that the fear responses to the prepared stimuli were much more resistant to extinction than were the responses developed to the guns and wires.[29,30]

Stronger support for this preparedness theory comes from a series of studies conducted by Susan Mineka and Michael Cook at the University of Wisconsin.[31] These researchers demonstrated quite convincingly that monkeys could acquire intense and persistent fears of snakes through vicarious or observational conditioning. The subject monkeys, who were born in captivity and had never before seen a snake, were allowed to observe another monkey showing fear when exposed to a snake. Only a few minutes of the naive monkey's observing the other monkey demonstrate fear in the presence of the snake was sufficient to develop a full-blown snake phobia in the previously nonfearful monkeys. In a second study, another group of naive monkeys observed monkeys display fear in the presence of snakes (live and rubber toy) and flowers. Again, the observer monkeys rapidly developed fear reactions to both the live and toy snakes but failed to develop fear responses to flowers. It appears as if this rapid vicarious fear conditioning occurs to snakes, which presumably they are prepared to fear, but not to flowers. These subject monkeys had never before seen either flowers or snakes.[32] Nevertheless, their fears developed quickly and persisted so intensely that they were undiminished at a later test three months later.

From the foregoing studies, the preparedness theory of fear development has received considerable support. Conditioned fear responses to slides of snakes and spiders are found to be more persistent than CRs to slides depicting neutral or other dangerous situations. They are not extinguished with repeated presentations of the CS alone and are not affected by telling the subject that no more shock will be given to them. And simple observation of fearful behavior by others is sufficient to cause intense and long-lasting fear in monkeys.

Whether or not subsequent research will help to clarify the prepared fear theory remains to be seen. Also, it is unclear whether or not such laboratory demonstrations of human and animal fear development can be used to explain human fear development under natural nonlaboratory settings. Nonetheless, the idea is intriguing, evidence is accumulating, and continued research should help to increase our understanding of the nature and development of human fears.

PSYCHODYNAMIC AND EXISTENTIAL/ANALYTIC VIEWS

The final two views or theories concerning the development of human fears and anxiety depart rather radically from the biological, conditioning, and informational theories previously presented. These two approaches to viewing fear and anxiety development are also different from each other in many ways. However, they share the position that the locus of anxieties is largely within the person's psyche rather than being developed primarily from inadvertent environmental exposures, such as conditioning, or from genetic endowments. The first of these positions to be described is the Freudian or psychoanalytic view.

Freud and Anxiety

The psychoanalytic position concerning the origins and development of fear and anxiety was detailed by Sigmund Freud during the 1920s in a book entitled *The Problem of Anxiety*.[33] Although Freud's theory has been revised and refocused by later analysts, the theme presented here is basically Freud's.

Freud saw anxiety as an innate, biologically based emotional state of displeasure. Anxiety itself was therefore a natural state. The experience of anxiety was seen as important in that it provided an occasion to learn how to deal with the vicissitudes of life. However, if the individual's early experiences were such that he or she did not learn to handle the inevitable anxiety appropriately, the result was the problem of neurosis.

Anxiety, according to Freud, is first experienced by infants at birth when they are rudely exposed to the intense stimulation associated with the birth process. Since the infant has not yet developed its personality, there are no means by which it can cope with the felt anxiety. It is the job of the parents to keep stimulation, such as hunger, within bounds. Another source of anxiety for the infant is that associated with the loss of its mother who at that point is critical to the child's survival.

Toward the end of the first year, the child begins to develop its *ego*. The ego's task is to mediate the biological urges and needs of the *id* (the inborn, animalistic portion of the personality) and the social or environmental demands of society, which, at this point, are represented by the parents. As the ego develops, it also learns to recognize potential threats to the individual. The anticipation by the ego of threats or harm results in what is called *signal anxiety*. Early sources of this signal anxiety generated by the ego's perception of threat included such situations as loss of a loved object and loss of an object's love (separation anxiety). Through the next few years, as the child develops, other sources of threat result in anxiety, including fear of injury to the genitals, which are a source of pleasure and comfort. This fear is later seen as *castration anxiety*. After the *superego* or moralistic portion of the personality develops, the ego comes to fear punishment by the superego if it lets the id go too far in seeking gratification of its desires. These various sources of danger, perceived as anxiety, are experienced at an unconscious level of awareness.

Through these early experiences of anxiety associated with the exposure to the demands of society and progression through the stages of psychosexual development, the ego and superego become more or less developed. In the relatively normal person, these structures are generally able to cope with the anxiety generated by perceived dangers or threats from the id. This coping is accomplished through the use of ego defense mechanisms. It is through these defense mechanisms that the ego defends itself against the anxiety associated with the id's incessant demands for immediate satisfaction of sexual and/or aggressive urges.

The ego defense mechanism most frequently used is *repression*. Repression works by keeping an idea or thought from becoming conscious so that there is no consciously felt anxiety. *Rationalization* is also used to keep the urges at an unconscious level. Here the thought or urge is made to appear quite rational and logical at the conscious level, but the person is really deceiving himself. The true thoughts remain in the unconscious which protects the person from consciously experiencing anxiety.

Projection is the process by which the ego consciously denies a problem or urge and attributes it to someone else. *Denial* is seen when a person consciously ignores dangers, perhaps rationalizing that tragedies only happen to other people. Again, the conscious experience of anxiety is avoided.

These and other defense mechanisms serve to handle the anxiety generated by id impulses in those individuals whose egos and superegos are reasonably well developed. However, a weak ego could result if a person's early developmental experiences were such that he or she had all immediate needs taken care of, seldom experienced anxiety, and therefore never learned to deal with problems. Later on, if id impulses threatened them, these individuals would be unable to keep the anxiety under control or to repress it effectively. They would then experience intense anxiety, usually referred to as *neurotic anxiety.* Moral anxiety results from an overly strict superego. If the superego is constantly threatening the ego with punishment for considering id impulses, moral anxiety is felt as *shame* or *guilt.*

Freud described three major forms in which neurotic anxiety could manifest itself. *Free-floating anxiety* is experienced as a chronic state of apprehension or anxiety where there is not a specific external object or situation to which the person is responding. This would be represented by the high-level trait-anxious person who continuously feels anxious. The psychoanalytic interpretation of this state is that this person is constantly fearful of being overwhelmed by id impulses that may cause him or her to do something that would be unacceptable to the ego. The fear of the id is, of course, experienced at an unconscious level. However, the resultant anxiety is felt consciously since the ego, being weak, is completely unable to defend itself against it.

Phobias are the result of similar processes as free-floating anxiety except that the anxiety response is more intense and focused on some object or situation. The phobic object does not represent a real external danger. The anxiety from the id impulse is controlled by detaching it from the real idea or situation that subconsciously generates the fear. It is then displaced to some other object or situation that is only symbolic of the real internal threat. Consciously, the real threat is then made less recognizable and the person can give a more or less plausible (rational) explanation of the fear. For example, a snake phobia might represent a fear of strong sexual impulses or a fear of being castrated. The anxiety is displaced onto the snake, which symbolically represents a penis; but such anxiety can then be rationalized since some snakes can be dangerous.

Panic attacks also result from strong, poorly controlled id impulses. The person experiencing an attack has an intense "rush" of anxiety which is not displaced or attached to other objects as in phobias. Rather it appears to come out of nowhere since the person is consciously unaware of the true source.

The foregoing summary of the Freudian position on the origins of fears and anxiety is rather oversimplified, but a fuller analysis is beyond the scope of this chapter. However, in essence, fear and anxiety are seen as stemming from unconscious impulses from the id, demanding instant gratification of its desires. To the extent that the ego is unable to repress or satisfy these urges in socially acceptable ways, they are consciously felt as anxiety.

An Existential View

An existential view of the origins of fear and anxiety is the final position to be presented. Although the existential view is represented by many writers with differing theoretical outlines, I will note some of their common themes. In doing so, I will draw largely from the writings of Rollo May who is credited with being the American founder of existential therapy.[34]

In many ways, the existential analytic view is a version of the existential view of human life and of psychoanalysis, although it departs rather radically at certain points. The two views are similar in that both hold anxiety to be central to a person's psychological being. However, they diverge on the issue of the person's ability to control his or her destiny. The psychoanalytic position holds that the personality is formed or determined at an early age, whereas the existential position holds that a person is free to make choices in the world and therefore is personally responsible for his or her existence. Also, most existential positions see the person involved in a process of becoming; that is, of continually changing, growing, striving for meaning and values in life.

According to May (1978) and others, values and what they mean to individuals are the core of their existence. When a held value is threatened, the person experiences anxiety. Since all values are vulnerable to some threat, everyone will experience some normal anxiety. Further, this normal anxiety is seen as a prime motivator of change and personal growth. Anxiety can therefore be regarded as constructive if it is confronted consciously, evaluated, and held open to change. This flexibility—openness for change or reformation of values—is the essence of self-understanding and growth.

If these new challenges that are signaled by anxiety are not confronted but rather are avoided and blocked by repression or other intrapsychic processes to keep them from the person's awareness, the result is *neurotic anxiety*. The person has narrowed his or her experiencing and has cut off self-growth possibilities. Anxiety is therefore seen not as a sickness but as a symptom of avoided possibilities or opportunities for change and growth.

Another term often used in existential analytic theory is *existential neurosis*. This term, popularized by Victor Frankl, is characterized in a person by a lack of an inner sense of self and of a meaning in life. From these voids come feelings of emptiness, worthlessness, and anxiety. Existential neurosis comes from a failure to experience life on one's own terms. Persons whose lives are directed solely toward satisfying society's demands or goals without creating their own personally chosen destinies are vulnerable to existential neurosis.

This overview of existentialist anxiety is a drastically simplified version of extensive philosophical writings. But the emphasis, as I have noted, is on the processes of experiencing and evaluating one's own values and goals in life. To the extent that these processes are blocked or unused, the person experiences vague, ill-defined feelings of anxiety.

The existential analytic position concerning the origins of anxiety is considerably less specific than the other theories presented in this chapter. This lack of a definitive focus, however, is derived from the tenet that each person has his or her own phenomenal world. Thus, to understand a person's fears and anxieties, we must attempt to view the world as that person does. The values and the meanings that person holds are the units of analysis. Therefore, it is considered impossible to target precise situations that will induce anxiety in all people.

SUMMARY AND CONCLUSIONS

In this chapter, I have provided a broad overview of several ways of viewing the origins of anxiety and fear. These positions included that there is a biological basis of fear. It is now well accepted scientifically that the tendency to react to certain novel situations with fearlike behavior is in part passed on genetically. However, what is passed on is a more general tendency toward being fearful rather than specific anxieties and fears.

Some fears and phobias are acquired by classical conditioning. Although there are many clinical examples of such processes, it is clear that many people who have fears never experienced the direct conditioning of their fears. However, vicarious or observational learning can be another source of these fears. We can acquire fears simply by observing others being injured or frightened. Many fears are acquired by these indirect processes.

The preparedness theory of fears integrates biological information with conditioning and offers an explanation of why it appears so easy for some people to develop fears of small animals. We are all biologically prepared to develop fears of certain animals that could be highly dangerous to us and to develop conditioned fear reactions very rapidly to such animals as snakes and spiders.

According to Freud, neurotic anxiety is the result of the ego recognizing potential danger signals to itself. These dangers come from feelings emanating from id desires and urges that the ego must direct to socially acceptable channels of expression. If a person's ego is not strongly developed, and thus unable to defend itself adequately against these impulses, the person can become overwhelmed with anxiety. This felt anxiety can take the form of free-floating anxiety, phobias, or panic attacks.

An existential view of the origin of anxiety holds that excessive anxiety results from unmet or unaccepted challenges to personal values. If a person does not consciously acknowledge anxiety and does not grow, change, and develop as new opportunities arise, a chronic state of anxiety results. Stagnation, rigidity, and loss or lack of meaning in life may result in existential neurosis.

REFERENCES

1. T. C. Schneirla, "Aspects of Stimulation and Organization in Approach/Withdrawal Processes Underlying Vertebrate Behavioral Development," in *Advances in the Study of Behavior*, Vol. I, ed. D. S. Lehrman, R. A. Hinde, and E. Shaw (New York: Academic Press, 1965).
2. Gene Sackett, "Monkeys Reared in Isolation with Pictures as Visual Input: Evidence for an Innate Releasing Mechanism," *Science* 154 (1966): 1468–1473.
3. Gordon Gallup, Jr., and Jack Maser, "Tonic Immobility: Evolutionary Underpinnings of Human Catalepsy and Catatonia," in *Psychopathology: Experimental Models*, ed. Jack D. Maser and Martin E. P. Seligman (San Francisco: W. C. Freeman, 1977), 335–357.
4. O. D. Murphree, R. A. Dykman, and E. Peters, "Genetically-Determined Abnormal Behavior in Dogs: Results of Behavioral Tests," *Conditional Reflex* 2 (1967), 199–205.
5. Gallup, Jr., and Maser, "Tonic Immobility," 335–357.
6. Alexander Thomas, Stella Chess, and Herbert Birch, "The Origin of Personality," *Scientific American* (1970), 350–357.
7. Jerome Kagan, J. Steven Reznick, and Nancy Snidman, "Biological Bases of Childhood Shyness," *Science* (1988), 167–171.
8. Ibid.
9. Malcolm Lader and Loretta Wing, "Physiological Measures, Sedative Drugs and Morbid Anxiety," in *Maudsley Monographs*, No. 14. (London: Oxford University Press, 1966).
10. Irving Gottesman, "Genetic Variance in Adaptive Personality Traits," *Journal of Child Psychology and Psychiatry* 9 (1962): 223–227.
11. Sandra Scarr, "The Inheritance of Sociability," presented to the meetings of the American Psychological Association, Chicago, 1965.
12. J. Shields, *Monozygotic Twins Brought Up Apart and Brought Up Together*. (London: Oxford University Press, 1962).
13. Svenn Torgersen, "Genetic Factors in Anxiety Disorders," *Archives of General Psychiatry* 40 (1983): 1085–1089.
14. Svenn Torgersen, "The Nature and Origin of Common Phobic Fears," *British Journal of Psychiatry* 134 (1979): 343–351.

15. David Barlow, *Anxiety and Its Disorders* (New York: Guilford Press, 1988).
16. John B. Watson and Rosalie Raynor, "Conditioned Emotional Reactions," *Journal of Experimental Psychology* 3 (1920): 1–14.
17. Stanley Rachman, "The Conditioning Theory of Fear Acquisition: A Critical Examination," *Behaviour Research and Therapy* 15 (1977): 375–388.
18. Stanley Rachman, *Fear and Courage*, 2nd ed. (New York: W. H. Freeman, 1990).
19. Douglas Bernstein, Ronald Kleinknecht, and Leib Alexander, "Antecedents of Dental Fear," *Journal of Public Health Dentistry* 39 (1979): 113–124.
20. E. Bregman, "An Attempt to Modify the Attitudes of Infants by the Conditioned Response Technique," *Journal of Genetic Psychology* 45 (1934): 169–196.
21. C. W. Valentine, "The Innate Basis of Fear," *Journal of Genetic Psychology* 37 (1930): 394–419.
22. H. B. English, "Three Cases of the Conditioned Fear Response," *Journal of Abnormal and Social Psychology* 34 (1929): 221–225.
23. Bernstein, Kleinknecht, and Alexander, "Antecedents of Dental Fear," 113–124.
24. Joseph Wolpe, "The Dichotomy between Classical Conditioned and Cognitively Learned Anxiety," *Journal of Behavior Therapy and Experimental Psychiatry* 12 (1981): 35–42.
25. Lar-Goran Öst and Kenneth Hugdahl, "Acquisition of Phobias and Anxiety Response Patterns in Clinical Patients," *Behaviour Research and Therapy* 19 (1981): 439–447.
26. Albert Bandura and Frances Menlove, "Factors Determining Vicarious Extinction of Avoidance Behavior through Symbolic Modeling," *Journal of Personality and Social Psychology* 8 (1968): 99–108.
27. M. E. P. Seligman, "Phobias and Preparedness," in *Biological Boundaries of Learning*, ed. M. E. P. Seligman and J. L. Hager (New York: Appleton-Century-Crofts, 1972), 451–462.
28. Ibid.
29. Kenneth Hugdahl, "Electrodermal Conditioning to Potentially Phobic Stimuli: Effects of Instructed Extinction," *Behaviour Research and Therapy* 16 (1978): 315–321.
30. Kenneth Hugdahl and Arne Öhman, "Effects of Instruction on Acquisition and Extinction of Electrodermal Response to Fear-Relevant Stimuli," *Journal of Experimental Psychology: Human Learning and Memory* 3 (1977): 608–618.
31. Susan Mineka, Mark Davidson, Michael Cook, and Richard Keir, "Observational Conditioning of Snake Fear in Rhesus Monkeys," *Journal of Abnormal Psychology* 93 (1984): 355–372.
32. Michael Cook and Susan Mineka, "Second Order Conditioning and Overshadowing in the Observational Conditioning of Fear in Monkeys," *Behaviour Research and Therapy* 25 (1987): 349–364.
33. Sigmund Freud, *The Problem of Anxiety* (New York: Norton, 1936).
34. Rollo May, "Value Conflicts and Anxiety," in *Handbook on Stress and Anxiety*, ed. I. L. Kutash and L. B. Schlesinger (San Francisco: Jossey-Bass, 1981).

The Prevalence, Assessment, and Diagnosis of Anxiety Disorders

In this chapter, I begin with an overview of the prevalence of anxiety disorders and how these prevalence figures differ according to gender and age. In the second part of the chapter, I discuss some of the procedures for assessing or measuring anxiety and how anxiety disorder diagnoses are derived.

PREVALENCE OF FEARS

Throughout their life spans, few people are immune to developing some form of specific fear or anxiety problem. Fortunately, many of our childhood fears diminish as we age and gain maturity. Unfortunately, other fears persist into adulthood, and yet other fears can develop at virtually any point in our lives. In one long-term and comprehensive study, Macfarlane, Allen, and Honzik (1954) found that of a group of children, studied over 12 years, 90 percent developed at least one specific fear during this period that was bothersome enough to be considered a problem.[1] Thus, even problem fears must be considered normal if they are experienced by the vast majority of children.

Although a majority of these childhood fears diminish as the child grows older, many are retained into adulthood. Jersild and Holmes found by interviewing a group of adults that 40 percent of the fears they had as children remained with them into their adult lives.[2] Similarly, in England, Marks and Gelder[3] found that among a group of adult patients seeking treatment at Maudsley Hospital in London for specific animal phobias, their fears had been with them for an average of over 25 years, having begun at the average age of just over 4 years.[3] Clearly, although many childhood fears come and go, others persist into adulthood and remain of significance.

As might be expected, the prevalence of fears of phobic proportions is not as great as it is for the more common fears that are probably accounted for by a majority of those in the studies just cited. In an epidemiological study by Agras and colleagues, the prevalence of specific common fears was found to encompass greater than 40 percent of the population of the Vermont community that was studied.[4] However, the percentage of persons in this study who were diagnosed as phobic was only 7.7 percent. Further, those whose phobias were judged to be severely disabling, such as keeping the individual housebound, included only .22 percent of those surveyed.

Two more recent national scale surveys found prevalence figures generally comparable to those of Agras. Uhlenhuth and his colleagues found 5.5 percent of the adult population to qualify for the diagnosis of phobia.[5] Yet another larger scale study reported phobia prevalence figures separately for each of three communities. These rates were 7.8, 9.4, and 23.3 percent.[6] The first two rates are similar to previous estimates but the latter unexpectedly large rate of 23.3 percent is difficult to explain. Unfortunately, the more recent survey did not evaluate prevalence of common fears as did the Agras study. Highly similar fear and phobia figures have been found in Canada as well.[7]

Overall from these epidemiological studies, clearly between 5 and 10 percent of North Americans suffer from a clinically diagnosable phobia.

Another anxiety problem of intensity equal to or greater than phobia is panic disorder. Various estimates of the prevalence of these anxiety disorders in the general population range from 2 to 4.7 percent.[8,9] Further estimates indicate that up to 14 percent of patients seen in cardiology practices are suffering with these anxiety disorders.

When the prevalence of panic anxiety is added to that of common fears and phobias, we see that a rather sizable proportion of the general population is directly affected by specific fear and anxiety problems. From the cited figures it does not seem unreasonable to conclude that as much as 20 percent of the general population suffers from some form of significant fear or anxiety problem. And, greater than 90 percent have, at some point in their lives, experienced at least one specific fear, but of lesser proportions.

The general prevalence rates just cited give us some indication of the breadth of anxiety and fear as problems. However, such general figures also obscure many variations that are important for a more thorough understanding of the distribution of these problems. Of particular importance is how the distribution of prevalence and incidence changes with age and how they differ for males and females.

Age Distribution

One of the most salient characteristics of the distribution of specific fears is their changing nature with increasing age and maturity. Knowing these general age norms or guidelines is important for determining which childhood anxiety-related behaviors are normal for a child of a particular age and which ones seem to represent an anxiety disorder like those described in Chapter 7.

As early as the first three-to-four weeks of life, fear is recognizable in infants. Sudden, loud noises or loss of support typically result in behavioral manifestations of fear, such as crying, stiffening the body, and diffuse body movements. Fear responses at this level are essentially inborn reflexes and are thought to be diffuse emotional reactions. From this rather rudimentary level of generalized fear, the number of stimuli to which a child responds with fear increases.

As children become more aware of their environment and those in it, the objects and situations capable of eliciting fear change. For example, fear of strangers emerges during the second half of the first year and increases in frequency up to and through the second year.[10] However, remember that these early fears are highly variable and are not shown by all children because the specific response may be dependent upon whether or not a familiar person is present.

After the first two years, and as children expand their horizons both in terms of physical and intellectual development, these initial fears of loss of support, noise, and strangers rather rapidly decline for most. However, other types of stimuli or situations begin to take on fear-promoting qualities. Most notable is the highly consistent finding that fear of animals shows an increasing incidence from around three years of age, and by four or five comprises the largest category of children's fears.[11–15] Jones and Jones provided one of the most vivid demonstrations of the age-related nature of these specific animal fears by placing children of various ages in an enclosure with a large harmless snake and observing their reactions. No fear was shown by children up to age two. But by ages three and four, caution and hesitation were evident. After age four, definite signs of fear were displayed. They noted that the signs of fear were even more pronounced in the adults than in the children.

As the child matures past the fourth and fifth years, often a slow decline is observed in the number of specific animal fears. It continues to decrease into the middle school years. However, new kinds of fears begin to emerge as children develop the capacity for active imaginations. These new fears involve more intangible or abstract objects or situations, including fear of imaginary creatures, monsters, and the dark.[16,17] For most children, the fear of creatures declines rather steadily and becomes negligible after ten or eleven years. Again, other types of fears and worries enter children's lives that reflect their more immediate concerns. At this point, fears associated with school and social concerns become more prominent, such as fear of taking tests, and shyness and worries over social relations.[18-20]

Although the information presented does show some rather consistent age-related patterns across the several studies, they must be considered only general trends, since all children do not follow clear patterns of the waxing and waning of these specific fears. Many of these fears decline with increasing age, maturity, and, presumably, experience. However, these trends of decreasing prevalence in general obscure the fact that some also persist into adulthood.

Persistence of Fears

As noted earlier in this chapter, as many as 40 percent of childhood fears persist into adulthood. Further demonstration of this persistence is illustrated in the previously mentioned epidemiological study by Agras and his colleagues.[21] These investigators noted three different patterns of prevalence and incidence of specific fears over a broad age range. They found the highest incidence of specific fear and phobia development occurring during childhood and typically reaching their peaks before age ten. The prevalence rates, which reflect the accumulation over time, or persistence, showed three different patterns. One cluster of fears represented by fear of doctors, medical procedures (injections), darkness, and strangers, peaked at about age ten. From there, a rapid decline in prevalence was seen during the adolescent and early adult years, becoming negligible by the sixth decade. A second pattern including fears of death, injury, illness, separation, and crowds showed a steady increase in prevalence up to age sixty, followed by a sharp decline. The third pattern involving fears of animals, snakes, heights, storms, enclosures, and social situations showed an increasing prevalence up to age twenty. From there it showed a more gradual decline over the next 50 years, suggesting that these fears tend to persist much longer than the others.

The more severe fears, phobias, and anxiety states also show age-related patterns. Consistent with the previously presented data concerning the onset of animal fears between the fourth and fifth years is the finding by Marks and Gelder in Great Britain that of a group of patients seeking treatment for fear of small animals, the average age of onset of the fear was 4.4 years.[22] Further, among their sample, they found none of the small-animal phobias to have begun in later life.

In this same study, other phobias were shown to have considerably later average onsets. For specific phobias involving heights and storms, the average age of onset was 22.7 years, but people were found to develop these fears at most any age. On the other hand, disorders such as obsessive-compulsive disorder, panic disorder, social phobia, and extreme shyness tend to begin on the average during the middle teen years. However, cases of panic disorder and obsessive-compulsive disorder are now frequently found in patients who are much younger (see Chapters 7 and 9). With some exceptions, agoraphobia begins, on the average, in the later 20s.

Gender Distribution

The population distribution of fears and anxiety is frequently found to differ for males and females. In general, and particularly from adolescence on, females express a greater number and a greater intensity of fears and anxiety disorders in general than do males. The few studies that have evaluated gender differences up to the early teens show relatively few differences between boys and girls in the number of specific fears and the percentage of each gender that expresses fears.[23] Macfarlane and her colleagues found that of those who had fears over a 12-year span, boys showed a slightly greater average percentage.[24] However, at ages three and thirteen, a significantly greater percentage of females were found to have problem-level fears. In another study, Lapouse and Monk interviewed a randomly selected sample of parents concerning their children's fears.[25] The results showed overall that girls were reported to have a greater number of fears than boys. In particular, girls had more fears of animals, bugs, strangers, and dirt. An important side note was found in this study by Lapouse and Monk. They observed that most of the data on the prevalence of children's fears were typically obtained from parents' reports of their children's fears. Consequently, one cannot be sure of the extent to which the mothers' biases and/or lack of knowledge of their children's fears distort the reports. They investigated this problem by interviewing a group of mothers and their children separately. They found that mothers tended to report 41 percent *fewer* fears for their children than the children reported about themselves. This finding would suggest that the prevalence of children's fears may be considerably greater than indicated by the previously mentioned studies in which parents were the sole informants.

When considering older children, gender differences in fear expression become more clear-cut. However, since the consistency of these differences varies according to how fear responses are assessed, they will be discussed separately for each of the three fear-response components.

Self-Report

For most fears, particularly those involving small animals and medical/dental procedures, females consistently report a greater number and more intense fears than do males.[26] For example, my colleagues and I found females to report a greater fear of dentistry at the middle school, high school, and college levels. Also, in a sample of adult community residents and college-aged subjects, females reported greater fear of blood, injuries, and the like than did males.[27–29] Similar findings have also been reported for fear of snakes, spiders, and mutilation.[31–35]

These feared situations in which females report more fear than males all have the commonality that they portend possible physical harm. In contrast, reported fears associated with social situations show little or no gender difference. In several studies, males and females reported similar degrees of fear and anxiety associated with speaking before a group.[36,37] Similarly, Zimbardo reported that the prevalence of shyness, which is related to social fears and anxiety, does not differ greatly between the genders, although he found a slightly higher prevalence of shyness in males.[38]

In general, although females report more fears than males, it is important to qualify this generalization by taking into account the type of situations that are feared.

Overt Behavior

Although fewer in number, the results of studies investigating gender differences in overt fear behavior roughly parallel those found for self-reports. Females have been found to be less willing than males to approach, touch, or pick up snakes and spiders.[39,40] However, in a study observing overt signs of anxiety while giving a speech—a form of social anxiety—no gender differences were found.[41]

In three studies that assessed fear of small animals, all noted an interesting gender-related relationship in the degree of correspondence between the subjects' verbal reports of fear and their avoidance behavior. Females' reports of fear were generally consistent with their demonstrated avoidance; that is, if they reported being fearful, it was highly unlikely that they would approach or pick up the animal involved. However, the males' behavior was less predictable from their level of reported fear. But in another recent study, my colleagues and I found that even though females reported more fear of blood, injuries, and medical situations, they did not report avoiding these situations any more frequently than did males.

Physiological Responsiveness

Although gender differences in physiological responsiveness in the presence of feared situations is somewhat consistent with results shown for the other response components, the relationship is less clear. The several physiological measures are each highly complex and do not always yield results that are clearly consistent even within a given subject. Consequently, relatively few studies have investigated gender differences using this component of fear responsiveness. Nonetheless, there is some indication that females exhibit greater palmar sweating in dental settings and report having fainted more frequently in response to blood and injury-related situations.[42,43] However, other studies report no differences for reactions to slides of spiders or of giving a speech.[44,45]

Clinical Fears

Since the data from the studies cited in this section come largely from surveys and other experimental settings, most of which relied on college students, the gender differences do not necessarily apply to persons with severe phobias who actively seek treatment. Nonetheless, the studies that report gender differences in patients who are seeking treatment are generally consistent with the research already cited. For example, in one report of a series of phobic patients, Marks and Gelder found females clearly to be predominant in a variety of phobias: animal, 94 percent; specific situations (storms and heights), 75 percent; agoraphobia, 87 percent; social phobia and shyness, 60 percent.[46] These percentages are consistent with other clinical reports of the gender distribution of phobic patients.[47] Interestingly, even with these clinical phobias, social anxiety and shyness showed the least sex differential. Other anxiety disorders such as panic disorder and agoraphobia, for example, were largely associated with females, whereas obsessive–compulsive disorders were closer to being even in male–female ratios.

Sources of Gender Differences

From the foregoing discussion of gender differences, clearly for most fears and anxiety responses, with the exception of social ones, females generally express more fear than males. This finding is most consistent in the postadolescent years. Although definitive explanations for these differences have eluded researchers, two lines of theorizing have prevailed. One line of explanation suggests that hormonal differences might play a role in the differential responsiveness.[48] A second, and somewhat more prevalent line, suggests that the observed differences are largely a function of gender-role expectations and training in which males have been expected to demonstrate masculine (fearless) behavior from early on in their social development.[49] Consistent with this observation is the fact that because of gender-role expectations, boys are typically encouraged—even forced—to play with and confront feared objects, such as small animals, worms, and the like. Most likely, through these direct exposures to potentially feared objects, their fears are diminished. This encouraged exposure is precisely the most effective treatment for overcoming fear and anxiety disorders. Young boys may be inadvertently immunized or "treated" for their fears as a normal expectation of growing up, whereas young girls are allowed, perhaps even expected, to escape from these same objects, thereby enhancing their fears. Although this explanation may not account for the full range of gender differences, there are enough examples consistent with this formulation to render it at least a partial explanation.

ASSESSMENT AND DIAGNOSIS OF ANXIETY DISORDERS

In the same way that each of us experiences fear and anxiety, we are assessors of anxiety as well. When we experience the sensations associated with anxiety, we do an informal survey of these sensations, noticing our heart-rate increase, feeling tense, and the like, and saying to ourselves, "I feel nervous." Or, when we say that "Joan looked jittery before her big job interview," we are essentially assessing our own or others' state of anxiety or fear. When we observe specific features of our own or others' behavior that are characteristic of fear or anxiety patterns, we may label that state as *nerves, fear,* or some other such descriptive label. The processes of psychological diagnosis and assessment of fear and anxiety are not really different, although, of course, the specific procedures used and the depth of involvement are typically greater.

Psychological assessment refers to the use of a set of procedures for describing, forming impressions, checking out hypotheses, and making decisions concerning a person's psychological characteristics and emotional states.[50] In general, the definition of psychological assessment can be readily adapted to the more specific concern of fear or anxiety assessment. Anxiety assessment involves the systematic gathering of information concerning a person's actions and reactions that fall into the domain of fear and anxiety responses. This anxiety-related information can be used to form clinical impressions, to describe the person with respect to his or her state or trait anxiety, fears, or phobias. When this process takes place in a clinical setting, it may lead to decisions concerning appropriate diagnoses and treatment. The two major methods used in anxiety assessment are the interview and the use of psychological tests and questionnaires. Examples of some questionnaires and interviews will be described in the following pages.

Anxiety Disorder Diagnosis

Diagnosis is closely related to, and follows from, the assessment. Diagnosis involves the determination of the nature and characteristics of a disease or illness by the process by examination and analysis; that is, by assessment. Diagnosis means determining a specific disease and differentiating it from other disorders. The specific anxiety disorders then are diagnoses. The interview and tests to be described are means of acquiring information in order to come to a decision about the specific diagnosis that best fits the person's symptoms.

The process of diagnosis involves identifying specific symptoms of anxiety that tend to go together into reliable patterns called *syndromes*. A syndrome is a collection of symptoms that tend to go together into a disease or diagnostic entity. The diagnostic or classification system to be described in the following chapters is based on the American Psychiatric Association's *Diagnostic and Statistical Manual of Mental Disorders,* currently in its third edition and recently revised. It is typically referred to as the DSM-III-R.[51]

In the remainder of this chapter, I will describe several methods of psychological assessment and the processes of diagnosis as applied to anxiety and its disorders. In the same way that fear was described as being composed of three components, these three components can each be assessed separately and each taken into account in determining whether a diagnosis of anxiety disorder is appropriate. These methods are grouped into assessment of the cognitive component, the physiological component, and the behavioral component. Some common anxiety and fear measures from each of these areas will then be described.

The Cognitive/Subjective Component

It has often been said that the simplest way to obtain information about how people feel or think is to ask them. This is the basis of the self-report mode of assessment. In the assessment of anxiety conditions, asking about a person's anxiety takes the form of structured interviews and various scales, tests, and questionnaires used to evaluate the components and the degree of the person's anxiety.

Interview

The clinical interview is the most basic of the information-gathering procedures. The interview provides an excellent opportunity for the person interested in fear or anxiety to acquire a broad spectrum of fear-related information directly from the individual that may not be obtainable by other methods. Among the types of information that are of importance in diagnosis and assessment that can be obtained in an interview are:

1. Descriptions of the situations under which the fear or anxiety reaction first developed
2. The frequency and specific circumstances under which the fear or anxiety response currently occurs, and where it does not occur
3. How the person responds when fearful, such as what thoughts run through his or her mind, what actions are taken, and what the anxious person is feeling
4. The effects of the fear or anxiety on the person's daily life

The areas noted here are related to those discussed in the first chapter as information used to decide if a given anxiety problem might be considered abnormal or not. Since it is impractical to follow the person around for days at a time and it is impossible to see what goes on in another person's head, our only entry into this important, but private, domain is through direct interviewing.

The interview can provide detailed information useful in the overall assessment and diagnosis. However, a free-flowing interview describing all that has transpired with respect to the anxiety problems, while interesting, could take one far afield of the most critical information. This lack of focus is why psychologists have devised the *structured interview* that allows the interviewer to focus on just those specific areas in question that are particularly important for the diagnosis. The structured interview ensures that all relevant information is obtained and that it is obtained in just the same way for each person being interviewed.

One widely recognized structured interview is the *Anxiety Disorders Interview Schedule–Revised* (ADIS–R).[52] The ADIS–R is structured so that the interviewer is prompted to ask specific questions that will elicit information required to evaluate the presence or absence of each of the anxiety disorders and to ensure that the correct diagnosis is obtained and that others are rejected. This is the process of differential diagnosis. In addition to assessing and diagnosing anxiety disorders, the ADIS-R also

TABLE 3
Anxiety Disorders Interview Schedule–Revised

Social Phobia
1. (a) In social situations where you might be observed or evaluated by others, do you feel fearful/anxious/nervous.

                                                                    YES   NO

(b) Are you overconcerned that you may do and/or say something that might embarrass or humiliate yourself in front of others, or that others may think badly of you?

                                                                    YES   NO

2. I'm going to describe some situations of this type and ask you how you feel in each situation.

Rate Fear and Avoidance

1	2	3	4
No fear/ never avoids	Mild fear/ rarely avoids	Moderate fear/ sometimes avoids	Severe fear/ often avoids	Very severe fear/always avoids

		FEAR	AVOID	COMMENTS
a.	Parties	____	____	_____
b.	Meetings	____	____	_____
c.	Eating in public	____	____	_____
d.	Talking in front of a group/formal speaking	____	____	_____

From: P. A. DiNardo, D. H. Barlow, *Anxiety Disorders Interview Schedule–Revised* (ADIS-R) (Phobia and Anxiety Disorders Clinic, 1988), State University of New York at Albany.

allows for the assessment of depression and trait anxiety. As noted previously, both often coexist with some of the anxiety disorders.

The ADIS-R is so structured that answers to its questions can be directly translated into diagnoses of anxiety disorders taken from the DSM-III-R. For example, Table 3 displays an excerpt from the portion used to diagnose social phobia.

Tests and Questionnaires

Questionnaires, tests, or inventories are the second means by which the cognitive component of fear and anxiety is assessed and are the method used most frequently for research purposes. Generally, these scales take the form of a series of statements or questions asking how the person feels, what symptoms and sensations are typically experienced, what objects or situations elicit anxiety, and what the person avoids because of anxiety or fear.

As noted in Chapter 1, there are many ways of categorizing fear and anxiety. Recall that there was state and trait anxiety, a number of types of specific fears and phobias, and seven specific anxiety disorders. In the following discussion, I will illustrate a sampling of the scales that are most often used to assess or measure anxiety, fears, and the anxiety disorders.

Trait anxiety is the term that describes a person's general, persistent pattern of responding with anxiety to a wide variety of situations. It is an enduring characteristic of the person—a personality trait. Consequently, the questions or statements that make up these scales are usually framed in general terms. The *State-Trait Anxiety Inventory* (STAI) is one of the most widely used.[53] The STAI is divided into the trait portion, referred to as *A-Trait*, and a state portion, called *A-State*. The A-Trait portion includes 20 statements relating to tension, anxiety, and upset, or their polar opposites. As shown in the sample questions in Table 4, respondents indicate how often each statement pertains to them *in general*, and the statement is rated on a scale from 1 to 4. Note that some of the items are reversed for scoring, such as "I feel pleasant" being scored in the direction of anxiety would be "Almost never."

The children's version of the STAI (STAIC) is called the How-I-Feel Questionnaire.[54]

A number of other available scales also measure trait anxiety, and even though they have different formats, they are all quite comparable to each other. Thus, a person who scores high on one will most likely score high on the others.

TABLE 4
Sample Items from the STAI-Trait Scale, Form Y

	Not at all	Somewhat	Moderately so	Very much so
I wish I could be as happy as others seem to be	1	2	3	4
I feel nervous and restless	1	2	3	4
I feel secure	1	2	3	4
I am a steady person	1	2	3	4

From: The State Trait Anxiety Inventory, Form Y, by Charles Spielberger and Associates. Copyright © 1970. Reproduced by special permission of Consulting Psychologists Press, Inc., Palo Alto, CA. 94306.

Understanding the level of trait anxiety gives us some indication of a person's anxiety in situations and over time, and thus, is of particular use in assessing generalized anxiety disorder. However, such general scales do not tell us how the person would respond in specific circumstances nor do they necessarily reflect that person's state anxiety. To get to this more specific level, we need to focus on specific situations. Several *state anxiety* and *specific fear scales* are available to obtain such information.

One of earliest state anxiety scales was developed by Walk to evaluate the amount of fear experienced by paratrooper trainees when taking their first practice jumps.[55] To obtain the trainees' cognitively felt fear (state anxiety), Walk devised a numerical scale ranging from 1 to 10 and arranged it vertically on a sheet of paper in the form of a thermometer; hence the name *Fear Thermometer* (FT). Walk tested the FT by administering it immediately prior to each trainee's jump from the training tower. Each trainee made a mark on the FT to indicate how much fear he was experiencing at that time.

This relatively simple fear-assessment technique appeared to be a valid means of obtaining a person's fear level. Walk found, as would be predicted, that the greatest level of fear was reported on the first jump, with subsequent jumps being rated correspondingly less fear-provoking. Further, it was found that as the number of jumps progressed, there was a clear relationship between fear level and the number of errors made by the trainees. Those who continued to report high fear made the greater number of errors in their jumps and vice versa. And those who failed to pass the airborne training program showed more fear throughout the training program.

This fear thermometer technique was a simple means of obtaining a measure of the cognitive aspect of a person's fear and was also adaptable to a wide variety of different fear-provoking situations.

Another state anxiety scale, and one most often used for research purposes, is the A-State form of the STAI. This scale is laid out just like the trait scale that was previously described. It differs in that the respondent is asked to rate his or her feelings "at this moment." Also, most of the statements to which the subject responds are altered to correspond to immediate feelings. Sample items of the A-State scale are shown in Table 5.

The general nature of the state anxiety inventories, such as the STAI and FT, make them highly adaptable to assessing anxiety in a variety of situations. However, their generality also limits their usefulness in certain situations and for certain purposes. They must be administered at the time the person is experiencing the fear or anxiety. Consequently, by their design, they cannot be used to predict how someone would respond in a given situation that may be encountered at some time in the

TABLE 5
Sample Items from the STAI—State Anxiety Form Y

	Not at all	Somewhat	Moderately so	Very much so
I feel calm	1	2	3	4
I am tense	1	2	3	4
I feel comforable	1	2	3	4
I am jittery	1	2	3	4

From: The State Trait Anxiety Inventory, Form Y, by Charles Spielberger and Associates. Copyright © 1970. Reproduced by special permission of Consulting Psychologists Press, Inc., Palo Alto, CA. 94306.

future. State anxiety scales are not useful for assessment outside the feared situation.

To evaluate how fearful one might be before the fact, another type of assessment scale is used—the *Fear Survey Schedules* (FSS). There are several of these scales, each containing a list of a variety of objects and situations to which the respondent indicates on a 5- or 7-point scale of intensity how much fear each situation would cause them.[56] Table 6 displays several sample items from the FSS-II.

If one were interested in obtaining detailed information of a given specific fear, then the A-trait and FSS approaches are inadequate. The FSS provides only the opportunity for a single rating ranging from "no fear" to "terror" concerning a particular object. And a single item does not allow for clear specification of the various conditions and circumstances that might affect the intensity of fear of that object. For example, a response to the question "How much fear would a snake cause you?" may depend upon the size, color, and proximity of the snake, whether it was in an open field, in a cage, or loose in your house! The ambiguity of a single item or question such as this would be expected to affect the accuracy of such fear ratings. One person might interpret the question as pertaining to a live snake in a

TABLE 6
Sample Items of Fear Survey Schedule II

1 = None	3 = A little	5 = Much	7 = Terror
2 = Very little	4 = Some	6 = Very much	

Being a passenger in a plane	_____
Blood	_____
Spiders	_____
Heights	_____
Closed places	_____
Snakes	_____
Speaking before a group	_____

Source: J.H. Geer "The Development of a Scale to Measure Fear," *Behaviour Research and Therapy* 3 (1965). Copyright © Pergamon Press, Inc.

field, whereas another might interpret it as a caged snake. Clearly, these two situations would result in different responses.

To address the problem of specificity and clarity of stimuli, a number of more detailed fear scales referred to as *specific fear inventories* have been developed. These scales can be used to assess in greater detail the various components of a potentially feared object or situation and the various ways in which a person might respond. Specific fear inventories have been developed for many of the more common fears and phobias and several representative samples will now be described.

The Dental Fear Survey (DFS) is a 20-item scale that my colleagues and I designed to survey various elements of three aspects of dental fear (see Table 7). The first area concerns avoidance of dentistry because of fear, asking the extent to which the person has ever put off making an appointment or cancelled an appointment because of fear. The second area assessed concerns the person's perceived physiological responses during a typical dental appointment, such as changes in breathing, sweating, heart rate, and the like. In the third assessed area the respondent is asked how much fear or anxiety is experienced during specific aspects of dental treatment such as when in the waiting room, when the dentist gives an injection of local anesthetic, and during drilling.

Studies using this scale have found that persons who score high prior to a dental appointment, indicating high fear, also tend to cancel more appointments, report more state anxiety when in the dental office, and give greater sweating responses during treatment than persons who score low.[57]

The DFS has been translated into several languages, and research shows that in cultures dissimilar from our own, such as in the Far East (Singapore), people show similar response patterns of dental fear to those found in the United States.[58]

The *Snake Questionnaire* (SNAQ), which is designed to assess fear of snakes,[59] is composed of 30 statements to which the respondents answer true or false as it applies to them. As with the DFS, these statements address the areas of avoidance of situations where snakes might be present, physical responses

TABLE 7
Sample Items from the Dental Fear Survey

Has fear of dentistry ever caused you to cancel or not appear for a dental appointment?

1	2	3	4	5
Never	Once or twice	A few times	Often	Nearly every time

When having dental work done:
  My muscles become tense:

1	2	3	4	5
Never	A little	Somewhat	Much	Very much

  My heart beats faster:

1	2	3	4	5
Not at all	A little	Somewhat	Much	Very much

How much fear do you experience when:
  Being seated in the dental chair?

1	2	3	4	5
Not at all	A little	Somewhat	Much	Very much

  When seeing the anesthetic needle:

1	2	3	4	5
Not at all	A little	Somewhat	Much	Very much

Source: Kleinknecht *et al.* Copyright © 1975.

felt while in the presence of a snake, and thoughts a person might have about snakes. Table 8 shows some sample items from the SNAQ.

The Maudsley Obsessional-Compulsive Inventory (MOC) was developed to assess the extent and type of obsessive and com-

TABLE 8
Sample Items from SNAQ

	True	False
I avoid going to parks or on camping trips because there may be snakes about.	___	___
I shudder when I think of snakes.	___	___
Some snakes are very attractive to look at.	___	___
I enjoy watching snakes at the zoo.	___	___

Source: Klorman *et al.* Psychometric Description of Some Specific Fear Questionnaires, *Behavior Therapy* 5 (1974): 401–409. Copyright © 1974 by Academic Press, Inc.

pulsive behaviors and symptoms a person might exhibit.[60] The MOC is composed of 30 true-false questions, such as "I frequently have to check things several times" and "I avoid using public telephones because of possible contamination." This inventory allows for a total score of "obsessiveness" and is further separated into four subscales to assess the various types of obsessive and compulsive behavior and thinking patterns, including checking, washing, slowness-repetition, and doubting-conscientious.

The Physiological Component

Assessment of the physiological component of anxiety or fear involves the measurement of the effects of activation of the nervous system, particularly the ANS. In Chapter 1, the ANS was described as being composed of two divisions: the sympathetic division (SNS), which is responsible for energizing and mobilizing the body for fight or flight to meet threats, and the parasympathetic division (PNS), which functions to conserve energy supplies. The SNS was described as the system that becomes most activated during fear and anxiety. Consequently, psychophysiological assessment focuses on measurement of changes resulting directly or indirectly from SNS activation. Other portions of the nervous system also become involved and can be measured, including the electrical activity of the brain and of skeletal muscles.

Many of the changes in ANS activity are readily apparent to the casual observer. We have all observed others who, when under stress, display facial flushing, pulsing of arteries, pounding of the heart, and sweating. However, these casual observations do not lend themselves well to precise measurement. Further, many other ANS functions are not readily observable without special electronic sensing equipment. This equipment, the polygraph, allows for the simultaneous monitoring and continuous recording of minute changes in a variety of organ systems. Some of these systems and their measurements will now be described.

The Cardiovascular System

The cardiovascular system involves the heart and the extensive system of arteries, capillaries, and veins. For our present purposes, two measures of this system will be described: the heart rate (H/R) and blood pressure (B/P). Although these functions are affected by states of fear and anxiety, it should be clear that they are also affected by many other conditions and are also influenced by the brain and the many endocrines of the body. As a whole, the H/R is controlled by the PNS for its normal rhythmic pacing. Under stress or threat, the SNS becomes activated and inhibits PNS activity which results in an increase in heart rate.

The H/R can be measured in several ways. Perhaps the most common is the one we have all experienced at the doctor's office: taking a pulse by hand. The wrist is held to feel the pulsing of the radical artery and the number of pulses per minute is recorded. A more precise and informative measure of H/R is obtained by the *electrocardiogram* (EKG). The EKG is a recording of electrical activity of the heart muscles. Measured by electrodes attached to the body, the EKG gives a continuous record of heart muscle contractions or beats. The beats are then converted to beats per minute which can be read out on a polygraph or given as a visual display.

The normal heart rate for adults at rest is about 70 BPM. This rate, of course, fluctuates as a function of many conditions, including fear. When extremely frightened or panicky, a person's H/R can easily double the resting rate.

Blood pressure changes, also under the control of the ANS, are often taken as a measure of fear and anxiety. As with H/R, blood pressure is typically taken at the doctor's office. An inflatable cuff (a *sphygmomanometer*) is placed around the upper arm to cut off arterial blood flow. As the cuff is gradually deflated, the amount of pressure present at the time a pulsing is first heard using a stethoscope is called the *systolic* pressure. This is the pressure with which the heart is pumping and is measured in millimeters of mercury (mmHg). As pressure is released further, the sounds from the artery disappear. The pressure at this point is called the *diastolic* pressure, the pressure of the blood when the heart is at rest or between contractions. Blood pressure measurement is expressed as systolic/diastolic. The average blood pressure for adults at rest is 120/80 mmHg.

The Skin

A second common system of physiologic response involves electrical changes in the skin. These response properties of the skin are called *electrodermal activity* (EDA), referring to changes in the electrical characteristics of the skin. Another term previously used to describe these responses is galvanic skin response (GSR).[61] Changes in EDA are, in part, a result of changes in the vasomotor system (dilation/contraction of underlying blood vessels), electrical properties of skin tissues, and sweat gland activity. These measures of electrical activity of the skin are both directly and indirectly under control of the ANS. The sweat glands in the skin, particularly those on the hands and feet, are under the direct control of SNS. Changes in sweat content of the skin then affects the electrical activity since sweat, composed largely of salt water, is an electrical conductor.

Muscles

Although not directly controlled by the ANS, muscle tension often increases with fear and anxiety states as part of a person's preparatory response to deal with threats. Muscle tension is measured by use of an *electromyograph* (EMG). As a set of muscles become activated for use, the muscles contract. The electrical change in those muscles is recorded and amplified. As more and more muscles become involved with increasing tenseness, the corresponding electrical activity shows up as changes in the EMG, which is recorded on a polygraph.

Respiration

When fearful, a person's breathing rate may change, increasing the amount of oxygen supplied to the bloodstream and on to body tissues. Two basic methods are used to assess respiration rate (RR). The simplest method is to use a small thermometer, a *thermistor*, taped beneath the nose. The air being exhaled is warmer than that being inhaled. Changes from warm to cool as air passes the thermistor represent the number of breaths taken per time unit.

A second measure of respiration is somewhat more direct. A stretchable tube placed around the chest expands and contracts with each breath and exhalation. A device attached to the tube, called a *strain gauge,* can record on a polygraph changes that are due to the stretching. In addition to the rate, this device can also provide information about the depth of an inhalation.

Physiological response measures are very useful in assessing the extent of a person's anxiety or fear. When these physical measures are combined with the self-reported information obtained from the scales and questionnaires, they supply a great deal of information about the extent of a person's fear and anxiety responsiveness. To round out the picture more fully, assessment of the third fear component, overt behavior, should be included as well. Methods for assessing this dimension of fear will be described next.

The Behavioral Component

Direct observation of fear-related behavior comprises the third component of fear assessment. There are two basic forms of behavioral observation: (1) the *Behavioral Avoidance Test* (BAT), in which the degree of approach to or avoidance of feared objects or situations is observed, and (2) the *Performance Test*, in which signs of fearful behavior are observed while the individual engages in some fear-producing task.[62]

Behavioral Avoidance Test

As noted in Chapter 1, one factor defining abnormal fear is the extent to which it causes avoidance of objects or situations. Accordingly, we see persons fearful of closed spaces walking stairs to avoid elevators, snake phobics detouring around grassy fields, and those fearful of flying traveling by bus or train. Persons with agoraphobia typically fear leaving their homes, and if they do leave, they tend to avoid large public gathering places like malls and department stores. Such observations demonstrate the behavioral response component of fear. When such avoidance is extreme, it classifies the person as phobic.

To assess more precisely the behavioral component, laboratory situations have been developed in which fearful persons can be observed under standardized conditions. The prototype of this form of behavioral assessment was first described by Lang and Lazovik.[63] These investigators were evaluating the fear-reducing effects of *systematic desensitization,* a treatment procedure. To ensure they were assessing the full range of fear responses, they needed a controlled means of assessing avoidance of the feared stimulus: snakes. To do this, they placed a snake in a covered cage at the end of a room. Subjects were brought to the door and told what was in the room and that they would be requested to approach the snake. They were then asked to enter the room and to walk toward the snake as far as they were able. The actual distance from the door that they were able to traverse was measured to represent their level or degree of avoidance. If they were able to approach the cage, the experimenter asked them to touch the snake, and then to hold it. This same measure was then used before treatment to determine initial fearful avoidance and again after treatment to assess improvement.

The general procedures used in the BAT have been adapted

to assess a wide variety of fear-provoking stimuli. Similar situations have been constructed for spiders, dogs, and other small animals. Assessment of fear of heights has involved having subjects climb ladders, open stairways, and fire escapes. For agoraphobia, the therapist might simply observe the number of steps or the distance phobic persons can travel from their front door. Or for those who are more mobile, how long they can tolerate being away from their home. The BAT has many advantages in assessing the avoidance component of fears and phobias. It is relatively easily designed and administered, and can be adapted to many situations that are feared and avoided.

Performance Test

Once a person is in a given feared situation, other, more specific elements of behavior may be of interest that are not reflected in the BAT. Here we rely on specific behavioral signs associated with anxiety while the person is performing a feared act. For example, performance observations were used by Gordon Paul to evaluate effects of treatments for speech anxiety.[64] Paul constructed a list of 20 observable behaviors thought to be direct indications of anxiety. These behaviors formed the basis of his assessment instrument, the *Timed Behavioral Checklist* (TBCL). The presence of each of the behaviors was observed and recorded at periodic intervals while a subject gave a speech. The behaviors included such signs as stammering, clearing the throat, avoidance of eye contact, shaking hands, pacing, perspiring, and the like (see Table 9 for examples).

The sum of the number of observation intervals in which any of the behaviors occurred was taken as the behavioral index of anxiety. The same procedures of recording anxiety-related behaviors while the subject is either performing a task or engaging in a feared situation can be applied to virtually any situation. Other applications include adult and children's behavior at the dental office, social interaction anxiety, such as talking with members of the opposite sex (a form of social phobia), and being in the presence of feared animals.[65-67]

TABLE 9
Sample Items from the Timed Behavioral Checklist

Behaviors	Time Periods			
	1	2	3	4
1. Paces	___	___	___	___
2. Arms rigid	___	___	___	___
3. Hand tremors	___	___	___	___
4. Swallows	___	___	___	___
5. Breathes heavily	___	___	___	___

Source: G. Paul (1966). Reproduced with permission of the publisher. Copyright © 1966, Stanford University Press.

SUMMARY AND CONCLUSIONS

Nearly 20 percent of the adult population experiences fear and anxiety in one form or another to the extent that it can be a significant problem for them. The capacity to experience fear is innately present in all of us, being an inborn reflexive response to loss of support or of being startled. As a child matures, he or she begins to learn to fear certain objects and situations. Early on, children learn to fear animals and other tangible threatening objects. As they mature mentally, they develop fears of imaginary creatures. Still later when they are in their teens, their fears seem to center around social concerns with peers. Through most of this growing up, particularly beginning in the teens, females report and display somewhat more fear than males.

Fear or anxiety assessment was discussed as the set of procedures for describing, forming impressions, checking out hypotheses, and making decisions concerning a person's characteristic pattern of responses to fear or anxiety-producing situations. To assess these response patterns, measurements are needed to evaluate the relative levels of fear and anxiety.

To assess the cognitive component, the interview and paper-and-pencil scales were described. The interview, being a rich source of subjective information concerning how the person feels and reacts, also suffers from lack of standardization which, in turn, can affect the reliability of the gathered information. A sample of such scales was shown for assessing state anxiety, trait anxiety, and specific fears. These scales, however, have potential limitations owing to individual interpretations of questions.

To assess the physiological responses, electronic recording devices like the polygraph are often used. The various physical response systems most often used to evaluate fear include: the cardiovascular system (heart rate, blood pressure); the skin (electrodermal measures), muscles (electromyogram), and respiration rate.

The behavioral component is assessed by use of behavioral avoidance tests and performance tests constructed to directly observe how a person performs when confronted with specific fears.

REFERENCES

1. J. W. MacFarlane, L. Allen, and M. Honzik, *A Developmental Study of the Behavior Problems of Normal Children between Twenty-one Months and Fourteen Years* (Berkeley: University of California Press, 1954).
2. A. T. Jersild and F. B. Holmes, "Children's Fears," *Child Development Monographs*, No. 20 (New York: Columbia University Press, 1935).
3. Isaac Marks and Michael Gelder, "Different Onset Ages in Varieties of Phobia," *American Journal of Psychiatry* 123 (1966): 218–221.
4. W. S. Agras, H. N. Chapin, and D. C. Oliveau, "The Natural History of Phobia," *Archives of General Psychiatry* 26 (1972): 315–317.
5. E. H. Uhlenhuth, Mitchell Balter, Glen Mellinger, Ira Cisin, and Janice Clinthorne, "Symptom Checklist Syndromes in the General Population: Correlations with Psychotherapeutic Drug Use," *Archives of General Psychiatry* 40 (1983): 1167–1173.
6. L. N. Robins, J. E. Helzer, Myrna Weissman, Helen Orvaschel, E. Gruenberg, Jack Burke, and D. A. Regier, "Lifetime Prevalence of Specific Psychiatric Disorders in Three Sites," *Archives of General Psychiatry* 41 (1984): 949–958.
7. Charles Costello, "Fears and Phobias in Women: A Community Study," *Journal of Abnormal Psychology* 91 (1982): 280–286.

8. Isaac Marks and Malcolm Lader, "Anxiety States (Anxiety Neurosis): A review," *Journal of Nervous and Mental Diseases* 156 (1973): 3–18.

9. Robins, Helzer, Weissman, Orvaschel, Gruenberg, Burke, and Regier, "Lifetime Prevalence," 949–958.

10. Michael Lewis and J. Brooks, "Self, Other and Fear: Infants Reactions to People," in *The Origins of Fear*, M. Lewis and L. Rosenblum, eds. (New York: John Wiley and Sons, 1974).

11. H. Angelino, J. Dollins, and E. Mech, "Trends in the 'Fears and Worries' of School Children as Related to Socio-economic Status and Age," *Journal of Genetic Psychology* 89 (1956): 263–276.

12. MacFarlane, Allen, and Honzik, *A Developmental Study of the Behavior Problems.*

13. Jersild and Holmes, "Children's Fears."

14. A. Maurer, "What Children Fear," *Journal of Genetic Psychology* 106 (1965): 265–277.

15. H. E. Jones and M. C. Jones, "Fear," *Childhood Education* 5 (1928): 136–143.

16. Jersild and Holmes, "Children's Fears."

17. Stewart Agras, D. Sylvester, and D. Oliveau, "The Epidemiology of Common Fears and Phobia," *Comprehensive Psychiatry* 10 (1969): 151–156.

18. Jersild and Holmes, "Children's Fears."

19. Rema Lapouse and Mary Monk, "Fears and Worries in a Representative Sample of Children," *American Journal of Orthopsychiatry* 29 (1959): 803–818.

20. MacFarlane, Allen, and Honzik, *A Developmental Study of the Behavior Problems.*

21. Agras, Sylvester, and Oliveau, "The Epidemiology Of Common Fears and Phobia," 151–156.

22. Marks and Gelder, "Different Onset Ages," 218–221.

23. Maurer, "What Children Fear," 265–277.

24. MacFarlane, Allen, and Honzik, *A Developmental Study of the Behavior Problems.*

25. Lapouse and Monk, "Fears and Worries," 803–818.

26. Michel Hersen, "Self-Assessment of Fear," *Behavior Therapy* 4 (1973): 241–257.

27. Ronald Kleinknecht, Robert Kelpac, and Leib Alexander, "Origins and Characteristics of Fear of Dentistry," *Journal of American Dental Association* 86 (1973): 842–848.

28. Peter Milgrom, Louis Fiset, Sandra Melnick, and Philip Weinstein, "The Prevalence and Practice Management Consequences of Dental Fear in a Major U.S. City." *Journal of The American Dental Association* 116 (1988).

29. Ronald Kleinknecht and Joseph Lenz, "Blood/Injury Fear, Fainting, and Avoidance of Medical Treatment: A Family Correspondence Study," *Behaviour Research and Therapy* 27 (1989): 537–547.

30. Douglas Bernstein and George Allen, "Fear Survey (II): Normative Data and Factor Analysis Based on a Large College Sample," *Behaviour Research and Therapy* 7 (1969): 403–408.

31. Ibid.
32. Edward Katkin and L. S. Hoffman, "Sex Differences and Self-Report of Fear: A Psychophysiological Assessment," *Journal of Abnormal Psychology* 85 (1976): 607–610.
33. Ronald Kleinknecht, "The Origin and Remissions of Fear in a Group of Tarantula Enthusiasts," *Behaviour Research and Therapy* 20 (1982): 437–443.
34. P. D. Evans and G. Harmon, "Children's Self-Initiated Approach to Spiders," *Behaviour Research and Therapy* 19 (1981): 543–546.
35. Rafael Klorman, Theodore Weerts, J. E. Hastings, Barbara Melamed, and Peter J. Lang, "Psychometric Description of Some Specific-Fear Questionnaires," *Behavior Therapy* 5 (1974): 401–409.
36. Ibid.
37. B. E. Blom and Edward Craighead, "The Effects of Situational and Instructional Demand on Indices of Speech Anxiety," *Journal of Abnormal Psychology* 83 (1974): 667–674.
38. Philip Zimbardo, *Shyness: What It Is and What to Do about It* (Reading, Mass.: Addison-Wesley, 1977).
39. Mathew Speltz and Douglas Bernstein, "Sex Differences in Fearfulness: Verbal Report, Overt Avoidance and Demand Characteristics," *Journal of Behavior Therapy and Experimental Psychiatry* 7 (1976): 117–122.
40. P. D. Evans and G. Harmon, "Children's Self-Initiated Approach to Spiders," *Behaviour Research and Therapy* 19 (1981): 543–546.
41. Blom and Craighead, "The Effects of Situational and Instructional Demand," 667–674.
42. Robert Brandon and Ronald Kleinknecht, "Fear Assessment in a Dental Analogue Setting," *Journal of Behavioral Assessment* 4 (1982): 317–325.
43. Kleinknecht and Lenz, "Blood/Injury Fear," 537–547.
44. Katkin and Hoffman, "Sex Differences," 607–610.
45. Blom and Craighead, "The Effects of Situational and Instructional Demand," 667–674.
46. Marks and Gelder, "Different Onset Ages," 218–221.
47. Isaac Marks, *Fears and Phobias* (New York: Academic Press, 1969).
48. Fredrick M. Kopacz, II, and Barry Smith, "Sex Differences in Skin Conductance Measures as a Function of Shock Threat," *Psychophysiology* 8 (1971): 293–303.
49. Mathew Speltz and Douglas Bernstein, "Sex Differences in Fearfulness: Verbal Report, Overt Avoidance and Demand Characteristics," *Journal of Behavior Therapy and Experimental Psychiatry* 7 (1976): 117–122.
50. N. D. Sundberg, J. R. Taplin, and L. E. Tyler, *Introduction to Clinical Psychology* (Englewood Cliffs, N.J.: Prentice-Hall, 1983).
51. American Psychiatric Association, *Diagnostic and Statistical Manual of Mental Disorders*, 3rd ed., rev. (Washington D.C.: Author, 1987).
52. Peter DiNardo and David Barlow, *The Anxiety Disorders Interview Schedule-*

Revised (ADIS-R) (Albany, N.Y.: Phobia and Anxiety Disorders Clinic, State University of New York at Albany, 1988).

53. Charles D. Spielberger, R. Gorsuch, and R. Lushene, *The State-Trait Anxiety Inventory* (STAI) (Riverside, Cal.: Consulting Psychologists Press, 1970).

54. Charles D. Spielberger, C. D. Edwards, R. Lushene, J. Montuori, and D. Platzek, *State-Trait Anxiety Inventory for Children* (Palo Alto, Cal.: Consulting Psychologists Press, 1973).

55. R. D. Walk, "Self-Ratings of Fear in a Fear Invoking Situation," *Journal of Abnormal and Social Psychology* 52 (1956), 171–178.

56. James Geer, "The Development of a Scale to Measure Fear," *Behaviour Research and Therapy* 3 (1965): 45–53.

57. Ronald Kleinknecht and Douglas Bernstein, "Assessment of Dental Fear," *Behavior Therapy* 9 (1978): 626–634.

58. Peter Milgrom, Ronald Kleinknecht, John Elliott, Liu Hao Hsing, and Teo Choo-Soo, "Cross Validation of the Dental Fears Survey in a South East Asian," *Behaviour Research and Therapy* 28 (1990): 227–233.

59. Rafael Klorman, Theodore Weerts, J. E. Hastings, Barbara Melamed, and Peter Lang, "Psychometric Description of Some Specific-Fear Questionnaires," *Behavior Therapy* 5 (1974): 401–409.

60. Stanley Rachman and Ray Hodgson, *Obsessions and Compulsions.* (Englewood Cliffs, N.J.: Prentice Hall, 1980).

61. Peter Venables and Irene Martin, "The Relation of Palmar Sweat Gland Activity to Level of Skin Potential and Conductance," *Psychophysiology* 3 (1967): 302–311.

62. Douglas Bernstein and Michael Nietzel, "Procedural Variations in Behavioral Avoidance Tests," *Journal of Consulting and Clinical Psychology* 41 (1973): 165–174.

63. Peter J. Lang and A. D. Lazovik, "The Experimental Desensitization of a Phobia," *Journal of Abnormal and Social Psychology* 66 (1963): 519–525.

64. Gordon Paul, *Insight vs. Desensitization in Psychotherapy: An Experiment in Anxiety Reduction* (Stanford: Stanford University Press, 1966).

65. Kleinknecht and Bernstein, "Assessment of Dental Fear," 626–634.

66. Barbara G. Melamed, D. Weinstein, R. Hawes, and M. Katin-Borland, "Reduction of Fear-Related Dental Management Problems with Use of Filmed Modeling," *Journal of the American Dental Association* 90 (1975): 822–826.

67. A. F. Fazio, "Implosive Therapy with Semiclinical Phobias," *Journal of Abnormal Psychology* 80 (1972), 183–188.

Simple and Social Phobia

As mentioned earlier, Phobos was the son of Aries, the Greek god of war. He himself was as reputedly a fearsome figure, whose likeness was painted on the shields and weapons of warriors to cast fear into the enemy to frighten them away. We get the term *phobia*, which means "morbid fear," from that early mythical figure. Given this Greek legacy for our terms, it is only fitting that our earliest written descriptions of phobias should come from the Greek physician Hippocrates. Although Hippocrates did not use the term *phobia*, he gave us one of the first case histories of simple phobia with the description of Nicanor who became panic stricken at the sound of flutes when played at banquets at night. However, Nicanor was unmoved if he heard flutes during the light of day. Nicanor's phobia, like many today, was highly specific to only certain stimuli.

It was some 500 years later when the Roman physician Celsus first used the term *phobia* to describe an effect of rabies—*hydrophobia*, fear of water.[1,2]

Although such morbid fears had been described for thousands of years, it was not until the early 1900s that the term *phobia* came into common clinical use and everyday parlance. Since then, however, hundreds of different types of phobias have been observed, described, and named. The name given to a particular phobia is a combination of the Greek word for the object or situation feared and the word *phobia*. For example, *acro*, the Greek term for top or height, plus *phobia* becomes acrophobia, a morbid fear of heights. Table 10 lists a sampling of some of the phobias that have been clinically described. As can be seen, many of these phobias are highly specific and some seem to defy logic of how such a situation can come to elicit such intense fears. For example, how does one become dextrophobic or levophobic? What is there to fear from the right or from the left?

Phobias are intense, irrational fears that interfere with a person's life adjustment.[3] There are five basic characteristics that must be present to differentiate phobias from common fears. First, phobias are *persistent*. A person phobic of heights cannot be cajoled or talked into climbing a ladder, a tree, or a fire escape. Second, the fear reaction is *irrational* in that it is clearly out of proportion to any actual danger in the feared situation. Third, the individual *recognizes* that his or her reaction is excessive and unreasonable. Fourth, even with this recognition, the person has an overwhelming desire to *escape* or to *avoid* the feared object or situation. Fifth, this avoidance causes significant *disruption* or *limitation* in the person's normal functioning. It is this latter criterion that is the commonality of all of the phobias: fear-motivated avoidance that disrupts a person's life.

In this chapter, two of the three types of phobias will be described in some detail: simple or specific phobias, and social phobias. The third major phobia, agoraphobia, will be detailed in Chapter 5.

SIMPLE/SPECIFIC PHOBIAS

In the first chapter we noted that many people have fears and anxiety responses that may pose no particular problem under most circumstances. However, when conditions change, this previously latent fear can emerge and turn a person's life upside down, as it did Martha's.

TABLE 10
Simple Phobias

Animals
  Acarophobia; entomophobia—
    insects
  Apiphobia; melissphobia—bees
  Arachneophobia—spiders
  Batrachophobia—frogs
  Equinophobia—horses
  Ichthyophobia—fish
  Musophobia; murophobia—mice
  Ephidiophobia—snakes
  Ornithophobia—birds
  Zoophobia—animals

Natural phenomena
  Achluophobia; nyctophobia—
    night, darkness
  Acrophobia; hysophobia—
    heights
  Anemophobia—wind
  Astraphobia—lightning, stars
  Auraphobia—northern lights
  Brontophobia; keratophobia—
    thunder
  Ombrophobia—rain
  Potomophobia—rivers
  Siderophobia—stars

Blood-injury-illness
  Algophobia; odynophobia—pain
  Belonephobia—needles
  Dermatophobia—skin lesions
  Hematophobia; hemophobia—
    blood
  Pyrexeophobia; febriphobia—
    fever
  Molysmophobia; mysophobia—
    contamination
  Traumatophobia—injury
  Vaccinophobia—vaccinations

Social
  Aphephobia; Haptephobia—
    being touched
  Catagelophobia—ridicule
  Ereuthophobia—blushing
  Graphophobia; scriptophobia—
    writing
  Kakorrhaphiophobia—failure
  Scopophobia—being looked at
  Xenophobia—strangers

Miscellaneous
  Ballisphobia—missiles
  Barophobia—gravity
  Claustrophobia—confinement
  Dementophobia—insanity
  Dextrophobia—objects to the
    right
  Erythrophobia—the color red
  Harpaxophobia—robbers
  Levophobia—objects to the left
  Pediophobia—dolls
  Trichopathophobia;
    trichophobia—hair
  Triskaidekaphobia—the number
    13

Martha had become nearly confined to her new house. She, her husband, and her young child had recently moved to the new house located on a beautiful verdant acreage with a sweeping view of the valley. During the first winter and autumn, all was well. But by March Martha could leave the house only with considerable difficulty for fear that a snake might accost her. She could not let her child of 18 months out alone for fear that a snake might attack him. If she had to leave the house, she would grab her child, run for the car, and speed away before the snakes could catch her. While in the house, she was constantly vigilant for intruding snakes; she scanned the yard through the windows, and had dreams of swarming snakes. To make matters worse, the family dog regularly brought home dead garter snakes to lay at the doorstep. Martha could not eat fresh vegetables from the garden for fear that snakes might have touched them.

Martha was experiencing a simple or specific phobia. As is clear by now, the term *simple phobia,* as used by the APA's DSM-III-R, is meant to imply that it is a single, circumscribed object that is feared rather than that it is "simple" in the sense of being of little import. All of Martha's responses to snakes showed that she met all five criteria necessary for the diagnosis. Her fear of snakes was persistent, and her husband could not convince her that the snakes were harmless. Her response was irrational and excessive in that the small garter snakes were quite harmless. She did all in her power to avoid and to escape them and it prevented her from enjoying her home, from allowing her son to play; furthermore, she was preparing to give up her new house.

Although most people with a simple phobia have only a single one, research shows that certain fears and phobias tend to cluster together, indicating that some people with a certain phobia may have features of related ones. For example, a young moth phobic client I once saw had similar, but less intense reactions to butterflies. And the fears and phobias that appear to cluster often have similar onsets and causes. Most studies find the following clusters of specific phobias: small animals, blood and injury, and natural phenomena. There is also a large miscellaneous group of other, less common, specific phobias which are not included in these clusters.

Animal Phobias

The animal cluster of phobias includes fear of a wide variety of animals, the most common of which are dogs, cats, snakes, worms, spiders, birds, mice, fish, and frogs. Although animal phobias, and fears as well, are probably the most common in the general population, they are seen only infrequently in treatment clinics. It seems that either the disruption in one's life caused by these phobias is less than that for other phobias, or the individual can find means to avoid them in many cases. Martha's snake phobia had been with her as long as she could recall, but it had not been a life-disrupting problem until she moved and could no longer avoid the snakes without also avoiding her home. Further compounding this issue is the fact that simple phobics are typically highly embarrassed about their fears. They know their fears are irrational and they feel that they should be able to overcome them with "willpower." Agras and colleagues found that animal phobias accounted for only 4 percent of the phobics seen for treatment at the University of Vermont.[4] Similarly, Issac Marks reported that of the phobics seen at the Maudsley Hospital clinics in London, only 3 percent are animal phobic.[5]

Animal phobias have several distinct characteristics that set them apart from other phobias and indicate that they have their own natural history. They tend to develop very early in life. Marks and Gelder found that, in England, the average onset is at 4.4 years of age and rarely do they develop after the age of 7 or 8.[6] However, they can be acquired later if the person is exposed to some traumatic event associated with an animal, such as being attacked by a dog. Marks further suggested that the clear age-relatedness of onset indicates that there may be a specific age span within which children are readily able to acquire animal fears and phobias. After that age, it may take an unusually traumatic experience to cause an animal phobia to develop.

Also common to many animal phobias is that the fears diminish with maturation. A 5-year follow-up study of the phobics identified in the Agras community survey in Vermont found that of those under 20 years of age at the time of the original survey, 40 percent were symptom-free and the remaining 60 percent were improved after 5 years. However, those phobias that do not dissipate during childhood tend to persist. Of the phobics who are over 20 years of age, only 23 percent were symptom-free, 42 percent improved, whereas 35 percent were either unchanged or worse after 5 years. Although the particular study combined all phobias, the pattern of early onset with persistence over years is quite characteristic of animal phobias.

Significant gender differences are also evident with animal phobias. Recall from Chapter 2 that prior to adolescence, males and females showed few differences in prevalence of fear, but later, females' fears became more prevalent than fears in males. In adulthood, this differential remains strongly for animal phobics.[7] Marks reported that upward of 95 percent of animal phobics are female.[8]

Another characteristic of persons with animal phobias is that the phobias are generally highly circumscribed. In all other aspects of their lives, they tend to be as well adjusted as the population in general. They are no more trait anxious than others, and their fear is quite specific to the animal involved.[9] This monosymptomatic picture with generally good adjustment may be one of the reasons this group so infrequently seeks treatment. Seeking treatment is often precipitated by changing life circumstances that bring them in more frequent contact with the phobic object—as was the case with Martha. Similarly, John's circumstances changed quickly and brought his animal phobia to the fore.

John was a 26-year-old popular radio announcer who had a phobia of fish. In all other aspects of his life he appeared well adjusted. He was active, happy, productive, and well liked. Although he had the fish phobia as long as he could remember, he had hidden it from others because of his embarrassment over such a "silly thing." He simply found other things to do when family and friends went fishing, and, of course, he avoided fish markets and pet stores. However, he was moved to seek treatment when his parents invited him and his brother for a vacation in Hawaii. His brother was an avid scuba diver and had plans for the family to explore the underwater marvels of the beautiful reefs and tropical fish. The mere thought of coming face to face with a fish, especially on the fish's own turf, caused him to cringe and shudder. He felt his choice became one of not going with the family and giving up an otherwise great vacation, or facing the embarrassment of openly admitting his irrational fear.

John could live with his fish phobia under normal circumstances, but it became a significant problem for him when these circumstances changed. Further, his problem, although significant to him, did not severely limit his daily functioning as long as he could successfully avoid fish. Similarly,

Sally had feared moths as long as she could recall but had been able to get along without too great an inconvenience. As she got older, a number of things changed. She lived alone in an apartment and could not rely on others to chase the moths away. If a moth were in the apartment, particularly between her and the door, she would become immobilized and feel trapped. She would not allow the light to be turned on outside her apartment door since the light could attract moths. Living in a basement apartment and being unable to use an outdoor light was dangerous. These factors, along with the fact that she had become greatly embarrassed over her reaction in front of her friends, finally led her to seek treatment.

Although such simple phobias can be debilitating and even immobilizing for some, it is fortunate that they are highly treatable. As will be described in Chapters 8 and 9, such treatments as systematic desensitization and exposure can help the vast majority of those victims who are suffering from animal phobia.

Blood, Injury, and Illness Phobias

This constellation of phobias concerns fears associated with bodily harm. Within this group are specific fears of needles and other sharp objects, fear of receiving an injection, having blood drawn, being injured or seeing others with injuries, and fear of the sight of wounds and related situations. Often lumped into this group is fear of contracting some disease or illness. It is not clear at this time whether the fear of illness is part of the same constellation of fears as the blood and injury fears. Consequently, I will discuss both within this section but separate them where it seems appropriate.

Although the fears in this group are the more prevalent of the classes of phobias, they have been the object of relatively little research. Survey studies indicate that they comprise the largest number of phobias in the general population. The Agras community study showed that 3 percent of their population sample was diagnosed as having illness or injury phobia and Costello's Canadian study found 4.5 percent in a sample of females.[10,11] Among all phobics identified by Agras, 42 percent were of this type. Compared with animal phobias, these fears are also seen more frequently in treatment clinics. Marks reported that 15 percent of his series of phobics from Maudsley Hospital in London were of this type, whereas Agras reported that 34 percent of phobics seen at the University of Vermont Medical Center sought treatment for illness or injury phobias.[12] It is considerably more difficult to avoid blood, sharp objects, injuries, and the like, than it is to avoid a particular animal. Indeed, even hearing or thinking of their blood pressure's being taken is sufficient for some persons to experience intense fear reactions.

Since there has been less research on this group of phobias, the nature of the relationship among the several types is not clear. Consequently, I will discuss separately some of the specific phobias within the group.

Illness or Disease Phobia

This group is characterized by a person's being chronically anxious and worrying over the possibility of having some specific disease. Two separate patterns of behavior may result from this intense concern. Some persons may constantly search their bodies for outward signs of disease and overinterpret all seemingly odd sensations as indicative of their having the feared illness. They may also seek medical examinations often on account of this fear. Donald Goodwin noted that the specific illness feared seems to be whatever disease is most prevalent or popular at the time.[13] Currently, cancer appears to be the most popular, whereas in previous decades it was tuberculosis and syphilis before that. Persons with this phobic pattern who believe that they have or that they might contract a particular disease are often said to have *hypochondriasis*. These persons, believing that they *do* have the feared disease, who repeatedly seek medical confirmation of it, are sometimes called *disease phobics*, but their behavior pattern does not conform to the definition of a phobia, since they do not avoid the stimulus but rather seek information about it. Best to leave them under the category of hypochondriasis.

On the other hand, those persons who fear that they might contract a disease, and who thereby avoid all situations in which they believe they might come into contact with the disease, may more legitimately be called *illness phobic*. Persons with such illness phobias may also show a pattern of avoidance of doctors or of the self-inspection that is common among hypochondriacs. However, for the most part, avoidance is difficult since the feared situation may be something within the individual rather than an external object. Fear of doctors may also be a part of this phobia if the individual perceives the doctor as the source of confirmation of the feared illness.

Illness fear appears most prevalently among middle aged

and older persons, most often beginning after the age of 40. As with animal phobias, females appear to predominate with illness phobia, although the proportions are not as discrepant, with about two thirds being female, and one third male.[14]

Phobias of receiving *injections* also tend to cluster in this group as well as with blood and injury phobias (to be described next). In part, needle or injection fear is one of the reasons for fear of doctors and dentists. Many persons fearful of dentistry cite the local anesthetic injection as the reason they fear and avoid dental treatment.[15] For some, this needle phobia is highly specific as was the case with Jennifer.

> Jennifer was a normal 16-year-old teenager who was in need of considerable dental treatment. She knew and accepted that fact with little apparent anticipatory anxiety and came to her dental appointment with little apprehension. Once there, however, each time the dentist approached her mouth with the syringe to inject the local anesthetic, her arms would reflexively jerk up to protect her face. Each time this occurred she felt badly and said she would try not to do it again. But each attempt of the dentist met with the same protective arm movements. Jennifer's fear and reflexive avoidance of the needle was highly specific. She was not fearful of the needles in other situations. She regularly gave injections to her ill horse without even a thought of fear. Thus, it was not fear of needles but, more specifically, fear of needles being inserted into her mouth.

Fear of injections, like Jennifer's, appears to follow a pattern similar to that of fear of doctors and dentists, with onset being typical before age 10 or 11 with slowly diminishing prevalence to about age 60.[16] Information on gender differences for injection phobia itself are unavailable. However, for dental phobia, and blood/injury phobia to be described next, females clearly predominate, at least by their own reports.[17]

Further, fear of needles is one of the main reasons given for avoiding going to the doctor. In one sample of 200 college students, I found that 42 percent had either delayed going to the doctor or avoided it all together because of fears primarily of needles. Although many times illnesses clear up on their own, the potential for disaster is always present with such irrational avoidance. The next type of fear to be discussed is also highly related to needle phobia for many persons but involves an additional element.

Blood and Injury Phobia

Although grouped with illness and injection phobia, blood and injury phobias present a somewhat different picture from that already depicted. The apparently unique feature of persons who become phobic at the sight of blood and injuries is that the majority of them faint. For most blood/injury fearful and phobic persons, a biphasic response appears to be involved with an initial increase in heart rate and blood pressure, followed by a rather sudden decrease which results in the faint (see Figure 1).[18] This biphasic response is in sharp contrast to that seen in other specific phobics in whom actual fainting in the presence of the feared object is rare. Recall that the typical physiologic response in fear involves a sustained activation of the SNS with consequent increases in heart rate, blood pressure, and/or other systems. Fainting, on the other hand, is mediated by activation of the parasympathetic system, resulting in a decrease in heart rate and blood pressure. When the PNS is activated without the SNS to keep blood pressure sufficiently high to sustain blood-flow to the brain, fainting results. Fainting, of course, is highly adaptive when blood pressure is low, since when a person is reclined, the heart does not require as much pumping action to distribute blood throughout the body.

Because of the paucity of research on blood/injury phobics, little is known about them. Consistent with reports of the larger group of illness/injury phobias noted previously, females predominate.[19] In several studies of blood/injury fear and phobic among college students and their parents, my students and I found several interesting facts. Although more females reported being fearful of blood and injuries, they did not report any

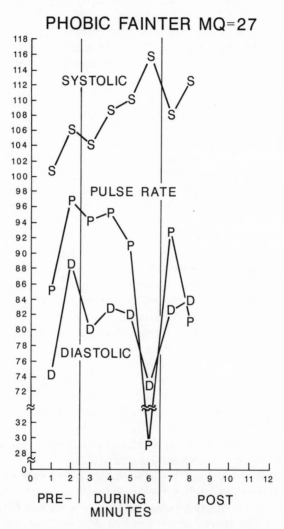

Figure 1. Blood phobic's cardiovascular reaction before, during, and after viewing injury on film.

greater avoidance of blood, injury, or medically related situations than did males.[20] As noted previously, simple phobias are often very specific and may be the only area in which the person has problems. Those who are fearful of blood and injuries are no more fearful of other frequently feared situations than are nonphobics. Blood and injury fear can be very specific.

In the same studies just noted, we gathered data on our subjects' parents' blood and injury fear as well as on their tendency to faint. There was no relationship between the parents' fear of blood and injuries and that of their children. However, a clear and unequivocal relationship existed between family members' blood and injury-related fainting. Sixty-five percent of our subjects who fainted had one or both parents who also fainted. In this case, it appears that fainting may be passed on, but fear was not. Our current interpretation is that the tendency to faint at the sight of blood and injury may be passed on genetically and the fear of these stimuli develops because fainting experiences are unpleasant and aversive.[21,22]

Much remains to be learned about this interesting group of phobias. For example, it is unclear whether the drop in heart rate and blood pressure, with the resultant fainting response, is truly unique to this group or whether it is simply an exaggerated response that nonphobics also have to a lesser degree when exposed to blood/injury stimuli.[23]

Like other phobias in this group, blood and injury stimuli are difficult to avoid. Who has not shed a drop of blood or seen someone else injured? Consequently, such a phobia can be limiting as it was for Jack.[24]

> Jack was a 16-year-old student finishing a technical school course in motor-mechanics when he sought treatment for his phobic reaction to blood and needles. He was concerned that his fear of blood and his subsequent fainting when he saw it would interfere with his work as a mechanic. Jack had fainted frequently during his biology classes at school and was about to begin a course of ambulance train-

ing required by the technical school. Fainting while working as a motor mechanic could be dangerous and, of course, an ambulance assistant who fainted at the sight of blood or injury would be of little use. Although Jack's reaction was clearly of a phobic nature, in all other areas of his life he appeared well adjusted and happy. It was also of interest, as is often found with blood–injury phobias, that Jack had three close relatives who also had this reaction, his mother, his brother, and an uncle.

Jack's fear had been disruptive to his education and his work. However, many such phobics have a potentially more dangerous consequence; they fear and avoid all medical situations.

Joyce has a blood- and injury-related fear that may have major adverse consequences for her in the future; she will not go to the doctor. Joyce reports that her fear and fainting episode began at about age 10 while at summer camp. A fellow camper attempted suicide by stabbing himself in the stomach. She saw the blood, got up, and immediately fainted. Since this experience, she avoids anything having to do with blood or injuries. Even friends talking of blood, the dentist, or cuts, initiates the fear and fainting in her. The specificity also is of interest here as Joyce is not fearful of needles as are many such phobics. Subsequent to the stabbing episode, Joyce reports having refused to go to the doctor to receive stitches for a gash in her leg. She now sports a large jagged scar. She has also refused to go to the dentist to have her wisdom teeth removed. Although these two incidents have not been life threatening, a future injury and avoidance could be.

Unlike fears of small animals, fear of blood, injury, and illness are virtually impossible to avoid. This is especially true for many of these phobics for whom even the thought of blood and, sometimes, merely feeling their heart beat can be sufficient to elicit fear and perhaps even fainting. The next group of fear stimuli, natural phenomena, are also quite difficult to avoid.

Natural Phenomena Phobias

The phobias within this group include primarily storms with thunder, lightning, and strong winds. Some investigators also find that fear of other natural phenomena cluster here as well, such as darkness, heights, and deep water.[25]

The only data on prevalence of these phobias come from the Agras study that found that 1.3 percent of their sample were phobic of storms.[26] This accounted for 18 percent of the phobias identified, second only to illness and injury phobias in prevalence.

The distribution of storm phobias over age groups suggests that onset is during childhood with a slowly declining frequency with increasing age. Two recent reports of small series of patients being seen for treatment of storm phobias are consistent with this age-related information. Lidell and Lyons found that 7 of their 10 phobics had onset at childhood, whereas Öst found 5 of 6 patients who were seeking treatment dated their phobias from early childhood.[27,28] It appears, therefore, that early onset is the typical pattern, but some can develop in adulthood as well.

In the three cited reports, all the persons identified as storm phobic were female. This predominence of females identified in adulthood with storm phobias is of interest from a developmental perspective. During the ages of 6 to 12, fears of thunder and lightning were found by LaPouse and Monk to occur in approximately 38 percent of children and they were equally prevalent among boys and girls.[29] Apparently the maturation and socialization process affects males and females differently with respect to overcoming their childhood fear of storms.

The prototype of this set of phobias involves fears of thunder and lightning. In many parts of the world, such a phobia can be severely debilitating, particularly during the summer

months. Persons with these phobias typically spend a great deal
of time organizing their lives in order to avoid being away from
home and being caught out in storms. They must arrange their
work, shopping, and outings to ensure that no storms are imminent. Typically, this includes continuous checking of weather
reports and calling the weather bureau for updated forecasts.
During a storm, their behaviors might include uncontrollable
trembling, crying, nausea, and rapid heart rate. Avoidance measures are taken as well, such as covering their head with pil-
lows, hiding in closets or basements, and the like.[30] This pattern
of fear-related behavior is well illustrated in a case report by
Doctor Lars-Goran Öst from Uppsala, Sweden:[31]

> This lady was 64 years old at the time she sought treatment
> for her fear of thunderstorms. She apparently had acquired
> her fear vicariously as a child. She recalled her parents be-
> ing very fearful when a thunderstorm arose and took ex-
> traordinary precautions when a storm was forecast. As an
> adult she was unable to stay alone in her summer house or
> to enjoy being outside during the summer because a thun-
> derstorm might arise. Her thoughts centered on thunder
> and lightning and [she] constantly checked the radio and
> TV weather forecasts. When a storm did come, she paced
> incessantly, was exceedingly anxious, had headaches, pal-
> pitation and an urge to urinate.

The overview of the different types of simple or specific
phobias illustrates many of their defining features, such as the
fearful and catastrophic thoughts, the increased physiological
responses associated with the fight-or-flight syndrome, and the
avoidance of these situations whenever possible. Hundreds of
other miscellaneous phobias have been described as well but do
not fit into these categories. Some interesting phobias stretch
the imagination to explain their occurrence. For example, how
does one learn to fear the sound of bathwater running down the
drain or fear a three-legged stool?[32]
The class of phobias to which we now turn are not so diffi-

cult to comprehend because we all can empathize to some extent with the fears associated with other people—social phobias.

SOCIAL PHOBIAS

Social phobias involve fears associated with other people which do not necessarily include fears of specific individuals *per se*; rather the essential element of the several social phobias is that the individual feels that he or she is the object of scrutiny by others. These phobias involve an intense fear of being observed and a fear that one is being, or might be, evaluated by other persons. The fear of observation and evaluation also involves fear of being humiliated and embarrassed. Although there is a relatively circumscribed situation to which social phobics react, such as public speaking, the phobia can take on broad and highly limiting proportions. It is very difficult to avoid being seen by other people.

As with the simple phobia, Hippocrates is credited with providing one of the first case accounts of a social phobia. Robert Burton's 1621 volume, *Anatomy of Melancholy,* includes the following quote attributed to Hippocrates:[33]

> through bashfulness, suspicion, and timorousness, will not be seen abroad; . . . He dare not come in company, for fear he should be misused, disgraced, overshoot himself in gesture or speeches, or be sick; he thinks every man observes him. . . . (p. 272)

Further, no class of people, mortal or immortal, is spared this affliction. Burton tells us that even the gods were susceptible to such conditions: "Jupiter so much afraid of his auditory, when he made a speech to the rest of the gods, that he could not utter a ready word, but he was compelled to use Mercury's help in prompting" (page 172).

A variety of specific social situations may become the focus for a social phobia. Among the more common types of situations are: meeting strangers, speaking or performing in public, meeting authorities, being criticized or observed while working, using public lavatories or dressing rooms, eating in public, vomiting, blushing, or fainting in public, and writing one's name while others observe. Another variation of social phobia, called *generalized type* appears to be more severe. In the generalized social phobia the person fears all or almost all social situations rather than just one of the more discrete types noted previously.[34] In each case, the central issue is the fear that others will observe and negatively evaluate some aspect of the phobic individual. In most instances, the anticipatory anxiety of these individuals over what *might* happen if they actually enter the feared situation leads them to avoid the situation altogether. And, if they are somehow forced to enter the situation, they are so anxious that often their expectation brings about a self-fulfilling prophecy. Their anticipatory anxiety renders them unable to perform as they would like and, indeed, they may bring attention to themselves just as they had feared.

Some feared situations such as public speaking are common and relatively easy for most persons to avoid without significant restrictions in their lives. However, for others, this fear can be a significant hindrance to advancement in their careers; for example, if promotion to higher levels of responsibility requires giving speeches or presentations.

Estimates of the prevalence of social phobia run between 1 and 2 percent of the adult population of the United States.[35] As noted in Chapter 2, the social anxiety and shyness are relatively common, but such fears of phobic proportions are presumably relatively rare. However, by the very nature of social phobia (avoidance of interpersonal situations), many such phobics may literally be hiding in the closet. Among phobics in the Maudsley Hospital services, social phobia accounted for only 8 percent of those seeking treatment.[36]

Social phobics have a relatively circumscribed age of onset. Typically, the phobia begins in adolescence when teenagers are highly self-conscious and concerned with peer evaluation.[37] Occasionally, but less frequently, they begin after age 30.[38] In contrast to all other phobias, social phobia, like social anxiety, is more evenly distributed among males and females. Although females still appear to predominate somewhat, it appears to be the major male phobia.[39]

The following cases of *scriptophobia*, fear of writing in public, illustrate some of the features noted above. These case studies described by Biran involved three women who responded to a newspaper announcement of the availability of treatment.[40] For two of the women the onset of their phobias was during high school and for the third, when she was in her early 30s. At the time they sought treatment, the phobia had persisted for between 16 and 21 years.

All three women were unable to write their names in public, which resulted in none of them being able to write checks, use bank cards, or vote. All three had accommodated to their avoidance by arranging for their husbands to handle all financial matters that involved writing. Two had avoided even telling their husbands of their fears. As is usually characteristic of social phobics in general, they experienced less fear if they were in the company of a trusted family member. The more formal the situation, the more anticipatory anxiety and fear they experienced.

When anticipating or encountering their feared situation, they experienced physiological symptoms of heart palpitations, shortness of breath, trembling hands, sweating, and dizziness. When confronted with having to write their names, they said to themselves, "People will wonder what's wrong with me," "I feel clumsy," "People might think that I am not stable, that something is wrong with me."[41]

A social phobia like scriptophobia can be mightily frustrating for the sufferer, as it was for Pat. Pat was a 28-year-old woman whose scriptophobia cost her something she had coveted for a long time. She was engaged to a man of considerable financial resources who promised to buy her any car she wanted. Pat knew what she wanted: a Nissan "Z." She had the specific one picked out and all she had to do was to sign the papers to register the car in her name.

Signing, unfortunately, was to be a major obstacle. The sales' desk was located in the center of a large showroom where several people, including the salesman, were seated as they went over the various papers to be signed. Pat had feared this part for days, knowing that she might have to sign the papers in front of these strangers. She hoped she could manage it because she wanted the car very much. However, as it came time for her to sign the papers, she became more and more anxious. As the salesman handed her the pen to sign, Pat could tolerate no more, and got up from the table and ran out the door, leaving the others quite dumbfounded. She would not return and felt too humiliated to make any other arrangements to get the papers signed. As much as she wanted the car, the anxiety over feeling humiliated was the stronger motivation.

In each of the above cases, the women also experienced some anxiety when in other social situations, particularly if they felt they were being evaluated or observed performing some task. This more general social anxiety is often seen in addition to the reaction to the more specific phobic situation. However, it is not always the case, as illustrated by George's reaction that was quite specific: he was phobic of using public restrooms.

George, who was 42-years-old at the time he sought treatment, dated the onset of his social phobia to his junior high school days. Being somewhat slower to mature physically than his classmates, he was very self-conscious of undressing, showering, and using restrooms at school when others were present. Even after he achieved puberty, his fears of being observed while in a restroom, in particular, persisted. Although he had accommodated to his fear for about 28 years, it was bothersome, restrictive, and made him ashamed of himself for being so silly. The phobia was most pronounced at the office where he held a responsible middle-management position. He would avoid using the office restroom if he thought one of his colleagues was present. If he miscalculated and happened to step into the restroom when someone else was present, he would become weak-kneed, his face would flush, his heart would pound, and he would be unable to speak. This reaction became worse if he was about to relieve himself and someone else walked in. His sphincter muscles would constrict and he would be unable to urinate. His evaluation fear was that if he could not go, due to the constriction, the other person would wonder what was wrong with him. This anticipatory anxiety over wondering what others would say became part of the vicious cycle that led to his fear and, in turn, kept him from being able to urinate, further reinforcing his phobia.

In situations where he felt anonymous, George had less difficulty, although he still felt some anxiety. At home, or when he was clearly alone, he had no fear at all. His wife of some 16 years was totally unaware of his relatively circumscribed phobia. He was too embarrassed to tell anyone. The therapist from whom he sought treatment was the first person he ever told.

Cross-Cultural Variations

In Chapter 1, we noted that while anxiety and fear are basic human emotions and are therefore found universally in all human beings as well as in the rest of the animal kingdom, the form they take are often shaped by the particular culture. One anxiety-related condition that appears to be a variation of social phobia is particularly prevalent in Japan. This condition, called *tai-jin kyôfu*, is either a cultural variation of social phobia or is a separate condition similar to what in the West is called *social phobia*. In translation, tai-jin means a social contact where the exchange of words and glances takes place between individuals in the presence of others. Kyôfu means fear. Thus, this is a socially related fear. There is a slight difference, however, from the social phobia previously described. Tooru Takahashi of the Japanese National Institute of Mental Health relates that persons with tai-jin kyôfu fear that they will somehow offend another person by some act or personal characteristic of themselves. For example, the most common form seen by Takahashi is the occasion in which the individual fears that he or she will blush (ereuthophobia) and that the blush will offend another person.[42] Also seen frequently is the situation in which the person fears that he or she cannot help staring at others and that this will make the other person feel uncomfortable. Other variations of tai-jin kyôfu include fear of giving off offensive body odors, giving improper facial expressions in the presence of others, shaking, being noticed to be perspiring, having a physical deformity, and having uncontrolled flatulence in the presence of others.

Until recently, tai-jin kyôfu was considered a culture-bound form of anxiety disorder in that cases of it had not been reported in the West. However, a case reported by Richard McNally and his colleagues at the University of Health Sciences in Chicago demonstrates that such cases may not be culture-bound after all.[43]

> Ms. M. was a 34-year-old school teacher in Chicago at the time that she sought treatment from Dr. McNally. Although she was initially referred for symptoms of obsessive-compulsive disorder, her own major complaint was that she avoided people for fear that she would embarrass them by staring at their genital area. Ms. M. had this problem only around adults, both male and female, but was not bothered around children. Further, she was most anxious in face-to-face situations but less so when the person's mid-section was concealed, such as when sitting behind a desk. As was true of the cases in Japan described by Dr. Takahashi, Ms. M. had a considerable amount of avoidance behavior. She avoided all social activities, face-to-face conversations, and she did not seek her masters degree for fear that she might embarrass professors by staring at their genital areas as they lectured.

Although such fears as Ms. M.'s are similar to social phobia in that the person fears that being observed will be the cause of a social problem, they do differ in that the person fears that he or she will be the cause of offending another person. Like the social phobic, the person with tai-jin kyôfu engages in avoidance of situations in which offense might be given to others. Also, like social phobias, tai-jin kyôfu typically begins in the mid-teens when the person exhibits the relatively trivial social improprieties of blushing or displaying stage fright. As the person reflects on the situation, it is built up far out of proportion until he or she comes to fear doing it again. Finally, as with social phobia, those situations in which it might occur again are avoided.

Another interesting characteristic of tai-jin kyôfu is its predominance in males. You may recall from Chapter 2 that social phobia differed from other phobias in that there was relatively little difference in the proportion of females to males. Thus, another cultural difference concerns which gender is most likely to be affected.

SUMMARY AND CONCLUSIONS

The simple and social phobias are probably the most prevalent of the anxiety disorders. Although they are not as crippling as some other anxiety disorders, like obsessive-compulsive disorder and posttraumatic stress disorder, the simple and social phobias can be quite debilitating as was seen with Martha's snake avoidance.

The roots of these two types of phobias may go far back into our primitive evolutionary past as suggested by the preparedness theory of phobia development. Although the depth of their ancestral roots may never be determined for sure, we do know that such phobias go deep into recorded history. Robert Burton's descriptions of ancient Greek phobics and the myth surrounding Jupiter's speech phobia tell us that the form and content of phobias has changed little across the past two to three thousand years. With some variation in other cultures, we still see the basic phenomena of irrational fear of nondangerous situations and fear of negative evaluation by others in most human cultures.

Simple phobias are the most treatable of the anxiety disorders with success rates approaching 100 percent when treated with the techniques described in Chapter 8. Some of the social phobias are highly treatable as well, but some are more treatment resistant. In the next chapter, the third type of phobia, agoraphobia, is described along with panic disorder from which agoraphobia is most often generated.

REFERENCES

1. Robert Burton, *The Anatomy of Melancholy*, 11th ed. (London: Chatto and Windus, 1907).
2. Paul Errera, "Some Historical Aspects of the Concept, Phobia," *Psychiatric Quarterly* 36 (1962): 325–336.
3. American Psychiatric Association, *Diagnostic and Statistical Manual of Mental Disorders*, 3rd ed. rev. (Washington, D.C.: Author, 1987).
4. Stewart Agras, David Sylvester, and Donald Oliveau, "The Epidemiology of Common Fears and Phobia," *Compehensive Psychiatry* 10 (1969): 151–156.
5. Isaac Marks, *Fears and Phobias* (New York: Academic Press, 1969).
6. Isaac Marks and Michael Gelder, "Different Onset Ages in Varieties of Phobia," *American Journal of Psychiatry* 123 (1966): 218–221.
7. D. R. Kirkpatrick, "Age, Gender and Patterns of Common Intense Fears among Adults," *Behaviour Research and Therapy* 22 (1984): 141–150.
8. Isaac Marks, *Living with Fear* (New York: McGraw-Hill, 1978).
9. Ibid.
10. Stewart Agras, David Sylvester, and Donald Oliveau, "The Epidemiology of Common Fears and Phobia," *Comprehensive Psychiatry* 10 (1969): 151–156.
11. Charles G. Costello, "Fears and Phobias in Women: A Community Study," *Journal of Abnormal Psychology* 91 (1984): 280–286.
12. Marks, *Fears and Phobias*.
13. Donald W. Goodwin, *Phobia: The Facts* (New York: Oxford University Press, 1983).
14. Agras, Sylvester, and Oliveau, "The Epidemiology of Common Fears," 151–156.
15. Ronald Kleinknecht, Rober Klepac, and Leib Alexander, "Origins and Characteristics of Fear of Dentistry," *Journal of American Dental Association* 86 (1973): 842–848.
16. Ronald Kleinknecht and Douglas Bernstein, "Assessment of Dental Fear," *Behavior Therapy* 9 (1978): 626–634.
17. Peter Milgrom, Louis Fiset, Sandra Melnick, and Philip Weinstein, "The Prevalence and Practice Management Consequences of Dental Fear in a Major U.S. City," *Journal of The American Dental Association*, 116 (1988).

18. Lars-Goran Öst, Ulf Sterner, and Inga-Lena Lindahl, "Physiological Responses in Blood Phobics," *Behaviour Research and Therapy* 22 (1984): 109–117.
19. Ronald Kleinknecht and Joseph Lenz, "Blood/Injury Fear, Fainting, and Avoidance of Medical Treatment: A Family Correspondence Study," *Behaviour Research and Therapy* 27 (1989): 537–547.
20. Ibid.
21. Ibid.
22. Stanley J. Rachman, *Fear and Courage*, 2nd ed. (New York: W. H. Freeman, 1990).
23. Öst, Sterner, and Lindahl, "Physiological Responses," 109–117.
24. William Yule and P. Fernando, "Blood Phobia—Beware," *Behaviour Research and Therapy* 18 (1980): 587–590.
25. R. Hallam and R. G. Hafner, "Fears of Phobic Patients: Factor Analysis of Self-Report Data," *Behaviour Research and Therapy* 16 (1978): 1–6.
26. Agras, Sylvester, and Oliveau, "The Epidemiology of Common Fears," 151–156.
27. A. Liddell and M. Lyons, "Thunderstorm Phobias," *Behaviour Research and Therapy* 16 (1978): 306–308.
28. Lars-Goran Öst, "Behavioral Treatment of Thunder and Lightning Phobias," *Behaviour Research and Therapy* 16 (1978): 197–207.
29. Rema Lapouse and Mary Monk, "Fears and Worries in a Representative Sample of Children," *American Journal of Orthopsychiatry* 29 (1959): 803–818.
30. Öst, "Behavioral Treatment of Thunder," 197–207.
31. Ibid.
32. Jerry Adler, "The Fight to Conquer Fear," *Newsweek*, 23 April (1984) 68.
33. Burton, *The Anatomy of Melancholy*.
34. Richard Heimberg, Debra Hope, Cynthia Dodge, and Robert Becker, "DSM-III-R Subtypes of Social Phobia: Comparison of Generalized Social Phobics and Public Speaking Phobics," *Journal of Nervous and Mental Disease* 178 (1990).
35. Jerome Myers, Myrna Weissman, Gary Tischler, Charles Holzer, III, Philip Leaf, Helen Orvaschel, James Anthony, Jeffrey Boyd, Jack Burke, Morton Kramer, and Roger Stoltzman, "Six Month Prevalence of Psychiatric Disorders in Three Communities," *Archives of General Psychiatry* 41 (1984): 959–967.
36. Marks and Gelder, "Different Onset Ages," 218–221.
37. Salvatore Mannuzza, Abby Fryer, Michael Leibowitz, and Donald Klein, "Delineating the Boundaries of Social Phobia: Its Relationship to Panic Disorder and Agoraphobia," *Journal of Anxiety Disorders* 4 (1990).
38. Marks, *Fears and Phobias*.
39. William Arrindell, "Dimensional Structure and Psychopathology Correlates of the Fear Survey Schedule (FSS-III) in a Phobic Population: A Factorial Definition of Agoraphobia," *Behaviour Research and Therapy* 18 (1980): 229–242.

40. M. Biran, F. Augusto, and G. T. Wilson, "In vivo Exposure vs. Cognitive Restructuring in the Treatment of Scriptophobia," *Behaviour Research and Therapy* 19 (1981): 525–532.

41. Ibid, 527.

42. Tooru Takahashi, "Social Phobia Syndrome in Japan," *Comprehensive Psychiatry* 30 (1989): 45–52.

43. Richard McNally, Karen Cassiday, and John Calamari, "*Taijin-Kyofu-sho* in a Black American Woman: Behavioral Treatment of a 'Culture-Bound' Anxiety Disorder," *Journal of Anxiety Disorders* 4 (1990): 83–87.

CHAPTER 5

Panic Disorder and Agoraphobia

PANIC DISORDER

A traveler in the woods, not sure of his way, begins to get an uneasy feeling. His skin feels odd, he begins to sense danger as his heart starts racing, and he feels sweat beginning to seep through his clothes. He is overcome with a sense that something terrible is about to happen, that he is dying, or that he is losing his mind. He feels like running but he does not know where to run. This terror mounts like an unbelievable crescendo. Seemingly, Pan has found another unsuspecting victim for his afternoon sport.

The seeming inexplicable nature of panic attacks has for aeons puzzled those who experienced them. This suddenness of onset, the intensity of the terror, the seemingly out-of-the-blue quality had to be attributed to something not of this world, something of the immortal gods. Since these attacks typically occurred out in the forest and fields, it was only logical that they should be attributed to Pan, the frolicking, mischievous, fun-loving deity of forests, fields, and flocks. Whatever the process by which panic attacks occur, they are still with us, just as they were described by the ancient Greeks.

Panic disorder is clearly the most terrifying of the anxiety disorders. Imagine having an intense attack of sheer panic or terror, not knowing what it is that you are reacting to. You see nothing that is frightening you. You can see nothing to run from, yet you feel more frightened than you have ever been in your life. This is what Tom was experiencing in the example given at the beginning of this book. Tom, and the millions like him, experience a whole host of symptoms, most coming from hyperactivation of the sympathetic portion of the autonomic nervous system—the fight-or-flight syndrome in full force. In addition to the intense physiological symptoms, panic attack victims feel as if they are dying or that they might lose control of themselves. Table 11 lists the typical symptoms experienced during a panic attack.

Each person having a panic attack does not necessarily have each of the symptoms each time. Often, they will experience, or recall experiencing, only a few. For an attack to be considered a full panic attack according to DSM-III-R criteria, at least four of these symptoms must be experienced. Fewer symptoms during an attack is called a *limited symptom attack*. In either case, the symptoms typically come on rapidly and reach their peak intensity within a very few minutes. The following case illustrates the suddenness and the devastating impact of the first attack.

> The first time it happened, she was riding beside her husband . . . taking in the rural scenery. It came like sudden death. . . . She couldn't catch her breath. She couldn't feel

TABLE 11
Panic Attack Symptoms

Tachycardia (rapid heart beat), palpitations	Dyspnea (difficulty breathing)
Fear of losing control	Chest pains
Fear of going crazy	Choking sensations
Dizziness/faintness	Parathesia (skin tingling)
Fear of dying	Hot or cold flashes
Feelings of unreality	Sweating
Shaking, trembling	Nausea

her heart beating. My God, was this a heart attack? Her mind screamed that she was too young to die. But she didn't die. She lived to relive what felt like death over and over again.[1]

Prevalence of Panic Attacks

The experience of panic attacks seems to be relatively common. G. Ron Norton and his colleagues at the University of Winnipeg surveyed adult evening college students and found that a surprising 34 percent reported having had at least one panic attack within the past year and that 24 percent had had one within the past three weeks.[2] Although there has been some question of whether all these students were reporting true panic attacks or whether they experienced phobiclike anxiety responses, these numbers do tell us that large portions of the adult population have experienced such frightening attacks. In a similar study, one of my students, Jennifer Lee, and I, using Norton's survey procedures, found similar results, while surveying panic attacks among high school students.[3] Clearly, from our research, although not all those students who indicated that they had experienced an attack had had a true panic attack, at least 11 percent of them had. For most of these students, the symptom profile reported was strikingly similar to that reported by clinical patients who were seeking treatment for panic disorder, and approximately 5 percent showed sufficiently severe symptoms to qualify for a panic disorder diagnosis. Subsequently, several other studies have verified the rather broad prevalence of panic attacks among high school students, college students, and the general public.[4,5] There now seems to be good agreement that somewhere between 9 and 14 percent of adults have experienced full-blown panic attacks. These figures are found in the United States, in Canada, as well as in Germany.[6,7]

Panic Disorder Diagnosis

Although as many as one third of adults and adolescents seem to have experienced one or more panic attacks, this experience is not the same as having panic disorder. As with the other anxiety disorders, the diagnosis is reserved for those in whom the anxiety is most severe and where it interferes with some aspect of the individual's life. To qualify for the diagnosis of panic disorder according to the DSM-III-R, the person must experience four panic attacks within a four-week period. In some cases, a single attack may qualify the individual for the diagnosis if they are so affected that their life is upset over constant worry that they might have another. Thus, if the impact of a single panic is so great as to influence the individual's life for some time, this, too, can be considered a disorder.

> Trevor experienced a series of panic attacks at age 26. Recently married, he was leaving town for two weeks to work a trade show in Dallas. His first day in town he was mugged, just around the corner from his hotel. The second day at the show, he began to feel ill, felt dizzy, his heart raced uncontrollably, he was hot and sweaty. After lying down for an hour, he felt better. This attack was on his mind throughout the next day but he seemed to be doing all right. After the show and a relaxing shower at the hotel, he was overcome by the dizziness again and his heart raced out of control. He called the paramedics, sure he had had a heart attack. They gave him a clean bill of health but encouraged him to have it checked when he got home. Back home an electrocardiogram and blood tests proved negative and he was given medication for panics. Again it struck at home with racing heart and dizziness the primary features. Paramedics again gave a clean bill of health. The fourth attack hit at home while he was relaxing in the back yard. Again the doctors at the emergency room found nothing but rapid heart rate and suggested that he might have eaten something bad. Another attack brought him out of a deep sleep at 3:00 A.M.

Although to Trevor, these attacks were of proportions that portended a serious, life-threatening condition, they were run-of-the-mill panic attacks. This is not to say that they were not devastatingly frightening. When a person's heart is racing at 150 beats per minute with no apparent cause, this is fightening!

Trevor's four attacks within a two-week period, each with greater than four symptoms, qualifies him for the diagnosis of panic disorder. Also typical of the onset of PD is the fact that the victim believes he or she is having a heart attack and the emergency room or paramedics are the first stop. Also, like other attacks, they tend to occur shortly after a series of stressful events, although often not during the event itself.

Types of Panic Attacks

Another consideration necessary for the diagnosis of panic disorder is that at least some of the attacks must be of the "spontaneous" type; that is, they must seem to come out of the blue with no apparent provocation, as described in Trevor's case. Trevor's attack came while he was at work, while relaxing after a shower, watching TV, and while asleep. Some investigators believe that such seemingly unprovoked or spontaneous attacks differ from those for which there is a more obvious stimulus. Donald Klein, one of the leading researchers and anxiety disorder theorists, has delineated three types of panic.[8] First, he includes the type that he calls *stimulus bound* panic, those that are clearly in response to phobic stimuli, such as animals or heights. Each time these panics happen the person is presented with the stimulus and never without the stimulus. These attacks, Klein believes, are more related to simple or social phobia rather than to panic disorder.

Klein's other two types are most specifically related to panic disorder and include the spontaneous or "unexpected" attacks that seem to strike without warning or cues. A related type Klein referred to as *situationally predisposed* attacks which are said to be more likely to occur in some situations rather than in others. But they do not invariably occur when the person is in the situation as with stimulus bound attacks of the simple phobic. For example, a panic-disordered woman might be able to enter a department store one day and proceed with shopping while experiencing only mild or moderate anxiety. Another day, however, she might have a full-blown panic attack while there. On yet another shopping trip she might be relatively relaxed. So, while she is more likely to have an attack while in department stores than at home, she does not always have an attack while shopping.

Where Do They Occur?

Panic attacks are not invariably tied to specific situations and, even when they are, they do not happen invariably. However, neither do they simply happen at random. Panics do seem to be more likely to occur in certain situations than in others. Although for most panickers, a majority of the day is spent at home, a small minority of panics occur there. The vast majority occur while in transport or when in public places.[9–11] Some of the most common specific panic sites include driving, particularly on expressways, bridges, or in highly congested areas; while traveling in public transportation like buses or airplanes; while in large department stores and supermarkets; and while standing in lines. It is as if these areas of high-intensity stimulation trigger the panic attacks, especially if the person feels overwhelmed and without a ready escape route available. Many panickers describe a feeling of being trapped. As will be described in some detail shortly, many people experiencing panic attacks develop strong avoidance behavior to ensure that they do not become trapped.

Although the majority of panics seem to occur under conditions of high-intensity stimulation along with feelings of enclosure, others occur in highly unexpected situations, such as while exercising, sleeping, and simply relaxing. Relaxing would seem to be a situation in which a person would be *least* likely to experience its antithesis—intense anxiety. This phenomenon, called *relaxation-induced anxiety,* has now become a well-documented occurrence.[12] The case of Trevor illustrates this phenomenon because he panicked after a relaxing shower, while relaxing outside, and while asleep. It appears that the change in bodily states from tension to relaxation may be sufficient in some individuals to trigger a panic attack. An explanation for this seemingly paradoxical phenomenon will be provided shortly when discussing the theoretical bases for panic disorder.

Who Has Panic Disorder?

Spontaneous and situationally predisposed panic attacks occur in as many as 14 percent of the general population. Of course, this many people do not experience a sufficient number of attacks to qualify for the diagnosis of panic disorder. Epidemiological studies conducted in the past few years indicate that between 1.5 and 5 percent of the adult population suffer at some time during their life from panic disorder.[13] Further, there is now clear evidence that females are more likely to experience panic attacks and panic disorder than are males by as much as 2 females to 1 male.[14] Although it appears that most panic disorder occurs in early adulthood (the late 20s to the early 30s), panic attacks themselves often begin considerably earlier. Examination of the data from large-scale epidemiologic studies of adults shows that the peak age group in which panics began was the group between 15 and 19 years of age.[15] These results, which were from adults who reflected on the time when their first panics occurred, might be subject to problems of accurate recall. Rather than asking adults with panic attacks when did the attacks begin, Jennifer Lee Macaulay and I went directly to ask a group of 660 adolescents about their ongoing experiences with panic. We found that the average age of a first panic attack among this group of teenagers was 13 years. As this group ages and more of them have attacks later on, the average will most likely fall into the same 15- to 19-year age group identified by Von Korff and his colleagues.

For many, it appears that panics begin to occur during the adolescent years. However, they do not all escalate into panic disorder. The typical age of panic disorder patients seeking treatment is in the 20s and 30s. Although this age scenario seems to fit for many with panic disorder, an increasing number of reports are found of panic disorder occurring in children as young as five years of age.[16]

Although a sizable portion of the general population experience panic attacks, there is evidence that they occur more frequently in some families than in others. Consequently, an individual who has a close relative with panic disorder is more likely to have panic disorder than another person who has no panicking relatives.[17] The only twin study to date in which panic disorder was examined found that if one identical twin had panic disorder, there was a five times greater likelihood that the co-twin also had an anxiety disorder than was the case for fraternal twin pairs.[18] However, in no case did both identical twins have just panic disorder. Somehow anxiety appears, in part, to be passed on through the genes. However, panic disorder as a specific disorder itself may not be a clearly genetic disorder, although the tendency toward experiencing anxiety and panic may well be genetically related. Although some portion of the cause of panic attacks seems to have a genetic contribution, the consequences of these attacks are learned patterns of behavioral avoidance called *agoraphobia*.

AGORAPHOBIA

The vast majority of panic-disordered patients live in some degree of fear of having another attack. Typically, this fear leads the person to avoid places or situations that they perceive as being similar to those in which they have had, or think they might have, a panic attack. This avoidance of possible panic-eliciting situations is called *agoraphobia*. According to the DSM-III-R, when patients are given the diagnosis of panic disorder, they are also evaluated for the degree of agoraphobic avoidance. The extent of the avoidance, if present, is rated as Mild, Moderate, or Severe. Although all panic-disordered persons do not exhibit such avoidance, the vast majority of those who seek treatment have at least mild avoidance.[19] As complex and as difficult as panic disorder is for a person, the phobic avoidance that so often accompanies it seriously compounds the problems.

The term *agoraphobia* has often been called fear of "open spaces." Literally, agoraphobia means fear of the "agora," the Greek word for marketplace. The term *agoraphobia* was first used by the nineteenth century German psychiatrist Karl Westphal in his clinical description of three men who were unable to walk across streets or such public places as the platz. These gentlemen experienced dread fear when they entered streets, particularly when the streets were deserted. They experienced dread when they were in the middle of the platz and thus felt compelled to stay close to the buildings that surrounded the square. They became highly anxious and dizzy when they ventured out alone. Being in the company of a friend or even carrying a cane or some such familiar object would ease the panic. Wine or beer helped as well. So, to some extent, even today, fear of the marketplace is an accurate description since shopping malls, department stores, and crowds, in general, are some common situations that are highly avoided by the agoraphobic person. Fear of open spaces is less accurate although some certainly fear being out alone. As will be described in greater detail, the major fear of the agoraphobic is fear of having another panic attack. They believe that if they venture too far from home or from other "safe" places and people, they might have another panic attack. Thus, the primary theme of the agoraphobic is the "fear of fear" or, as it is sometimes called, *phobophobia*.[20]

In its more severe form, agoraphobia leaves the person virtually housebound. Since their fear is so intense and pervasive, they cannot venture past their front door unless accompanied by a trusted companion, as was seen with Westphal's cases, and then only with considerable apprehension.

Although one can list an extensive number of situations that are feared and avoided by the agoraphobic, agoraphobia is not simply multiple fears or phobias. The central core for at least the majority is that they fear having another attack.

Progression from Panic to Agoraphobia

A common progression for the development of agoraphobic avoidance begins with an intense panic attack, which may take place while driving, for example. A man may feel his heart racing, palpitating; profuse sweating may occur, especially on the hands and feet. There is a sense that something dreadful is happening, that he is dying, going crazy, and may lose control of himself and the car. The first self-diagnosis is often that he is having a heart attack. He heads straight for medical help at the hospital emergency room where the physician's examination proves totally negative. No heart irregularities; no heart attack. He is released, told it was just "nerves," and that he should take it easy, maybe take some "nerve pills" or tranquilizers.

The situations in which the attack first occurred show a common theme as well. They typically occur in situations in which the person is physically confined or restricted: traveling by bus, airplane, or driving a car on freeways and bridges; being in enclosed places, such as elevators, theaters, churches, or restaurants. The feeling of being trapped with no escape available appears to be the common denominator of the circumstances in which the attack first occurs as well as the precipitant of later attacks and subsequently of situations to be avoided.

Such a frighteningly intense experience is not easily forgotten. The person worries about having another one, especially when driving in situations that remind him of the first attack; he begins to avoid those places. Then, perhaps, while waiting for a table in a restaurant, he is hit with another attack. He feels trapped, can't get his breath, and the same symptom complex occurs as before. He leaves without eating, and feels considerably better when he gets outside. Now he feels that he cannot go back to that restaurant nor to others for fear that it might happen again. After several more attacks in different situations, the safe territory becomes more and more constricted. As his options for mobility become more limited, he becomes a full-blown agoraphobic, confined to a few safe places when accompanied by a safe person. Agoraphobics most commonly report avoiding the following situations: leaving home alone, unfamiliar places, travel by train, bus, or airplane, crowds, large open spaces, enclosed spaces, shopping centers and department stores, movies, eating or drinking in public, crossing bridges or streets, and high places. This list leaves few alternatives for the agoraphobic but home. In many cases, the person may be able to leave home but only with a trusted companion, typically, a spouse or close friend or, in some cases, a pet. However, even when accompanied, the person will only be able to go to certain places. These places must be such that the phobic has a ready escape route in the event of another panic attack. If they were to go to a movie theater or church, they would take great care to ensure that they got a seat in the back on an aisle for ready escape if necessary.

This list of specific situations avoided should not be taken to suggest that agoraphobia is simply a compilation of specific phobias. Rather, these situations are elements of a relatively distinct pattern of fears that comprise a syndrome of its own.[21] Furthermore, in describing this syndrome, agoraphobics typically fear their reactions as much or more than the specific circumstances. The reactions that they fear include fainting and losing control in public should they experience a panic attack. Thus, it is not so much the situations that they fear but their reaction in those situations. The fear of reactions also have a strong element of social fears. They are fearful that if they should have a panic attack in public, they might faint or otherwise lose control which would cause them to be the center of attention. Other people will then wonder what is wrong with them and hence they will be negatively evaluated for making fools of themselves. It is in this sense that agoraphobia has been called *fear of fear*, or rather fear of the reaction which, in turn, may draw attention to them and make them subject to social evaluation.

Associated Problems of Panic and Agoraphobia

As if panic and agoraphobic avoidance were not enough of a problem, such persons are also found to be at significantly greater risk for other anxiety disorders and for additional psychological problems as well. Foremost among the associated problems is depression.[22] A large percentage of panic and particularly agoraphobic persons are found to show clinically significant levels of depression. For some, the depression appears to develop out of the seemingly hopeless situation of experiencing uncontrollable panics and associated phobic-avoidance patterns. For others, the depression may coexist independently or may have preceded the panic. Panic attacks are also relatively common among patients whose primary diagnosis is depression.

An article recently published in the *New England Journal of Medicine* by Myrna Weissman and her colleagues reported a startling finding: persons who experienced panic attacks and panic disorder are found to be at highly increased risk for suicidal thoughts and suicide attempts.[23] Even though it is common knowledge that suicidal thought and attempts are associated with depression, this is the first clear evidence that it is associated with panic as well. Furthermore, even though panic and depression are related, the increased risk of suicide attempts existed in persons with panic whether or not they were also depressed. Thus, the increased risk of suicide attempts has something to do with panic itself, over and above its association with depression.

In addition to depression, panic-disordered and agoraphobic individuals also are at increased risk for alcohol and other substance-abuse problems.[24] For many, the alcohol is one means by which they can control the intense anxiety they feel and allows them to venture from home, although in a less than alert state. Thus, it is a form of self-medication for the anxiety and panic. Looking at the relationship the other way, it is also found that anxiety and panic disorder and agoraphobia are common co-diagnoses in as many as 40 to 50 percent of alcoholics.[25] As with depression, it is not always clear which came first, the alcohol abuse or the panic. It may well work both ways, since as noted previously, alcohol can temporarily ease anxiety and panic symptoms, which can lead to its increased use as a self-medicant. Also, alcohol, consumed in addictive quantities over time, can increase anxiety and *cause* panics. Thus, there may be a spiral effect in that alcohol is taken to help the panic, but, in the long run, it actually increases the panic which leads to more alcohol to decrease the panic, and so on.

Stress Antecedents to Onset of Panic and Agoraphobia

It is now a well-supported finding in clinical research that, in the weeks and months immediately preceding the onset of panic attacks, panic disorder, and agoraphobia, the majority of patients experience one or more major stressors, usually in the form of a negative life event. Various studies found that between 75 and 91 percent of their patients had a recent stressor of this sort.[26,27] Typically, these stressors are of the type in which the person has experienced an interpersonal loss, endocrine changes from birth or pregnancy, or major illness or injury. It is as though these stressors accumulate and fester as they evolve into a panic attack. When it finally erupts, it is not uncommon for the person to be unable to identify the cues, since it seems to come out of nowhere as it did with Trevor. Of course, this makes it difficult for them to make the connection between the occurrence of the life stressors and the onset of their panic.[28]

THEORIES OF PANIC AND AGORAPHOBIA ONSET

The recent outpouring of research on anxiety and panic disorder has produced a bewildering array of information on the nature of these emotions. Attempts to consolidate this plethora of information into coherent theoretical structures have been productive and salutary. This integration of many seemingly disparate facts into a comprehensible, although admittedly theoretical, framework allows us to begin to understand the factors associated with the origins and the maintenance of these conditions. Current theories run the gamut of psychological explanations for the phenomena of panic to purely physiological explanations that imply that the panic-disordered person has something referred to as the "anxiety disease."[29] As a result, there is an assumption that there is something physically awry in the person that erupts periodically into a panic attack. More recently, the psychological and biological theorists appear to be coming together to integrate the data into biopsychosocial models that take into account the fact that those who experience panic attacks are, at the same time, biological beings with unique heredities, psychological beings with their own personalities, and social creatures steeped in the beliefs and values of the society in which they were raised. All these factors must be taken into account if we are to incorporate the many varied facts about these conditions. In the theoretical discussion that follows, I will outline two of the most current integrative theories of panic. The first to be described comes largely from a neurological perspective recently presented by Jack Gorman and his colleagues at the Columbia University College of Physicians and Surgeons.[30] His neuroanatomical theory, while neurologically based, readily accommodates psychologial information.

The second theory is proposed by David Barlow, Director of the Phobia and Anxiety Disorders Clinic of the State University of New York at Albany.[31] Although Barlow's theory has as its major focus the psychological aspects of panic, it integrates the neurological and genetic data that exist today. Thus, these two theories, although approaching the problems from different directions, become quite complimentary to each other and together can integrate a great deal of the current knowledge on panic and agoraphobia.

The Neuroanatomical Basis for Panic Disorder

As I described in Chapter 1, anxiety disorders at the most basic level are responses of our physiology. It is our brain and its various structures as part of the nervous system that ultimately determine how we will respond to any situation. To begin to comprehend the complexities of anxiety, we must look to the basic components of the central nervous system (the brain) that underlie fear or panic responses. The theoretical structure to be described is, by its author's admission, somewhat speculative,[30] but such integrative theorizing is necessary to generate testable hypotheses that can carry the theory to greater specificity and accuracy.

Gorman's theory attempts to integrate current knowledge about how specific parts of the brain are related to different aspects of anxiety and panic. The theory also describes how psychological influences enter in to stimulate these brain structures to respond in ways that we experience as anxiety and panic. This neuroanatomical theory begins by asserting that there are three distinct components to panic disorder: (1) the acute panic attack itself, (2) the anticipatory anxiety, and (3) often the phobic avoidance or the agoraphobic component.

The Acute Panic Attack

The acute panic attack is believed to originate from hyperactivation of structures in the lower part of the brain (the *brain stem*) at the base of the skull. This primitive but vital portion of the brain is essentially similar in all mammalian species. Thus, many theorists believe that all mammals at least and probably many lower species can experience panics. The brain stem is perhaps the neurological center of the fight-or-flight response and is where the signals emanate to elicit the physical symptoms of ANS activity, such as heart palpitations, stomach distress, breathing difficulties, and the like. Furthermore, through experiments, certain chemicals are now known that can artificially produce these symptoms in humans and in animals and do so by increasing the activity of structures within the brain stem. One of the principle structures within the brain stem that is directly involved in panic is the *locus coeruleus* (LC). This structure is the main center in the brain where *norepinephrine* or *noradrenaline* is used. Removing the locus coeruleus from animals renders them incapable of showing or experiencing fearlike behavior. At least one other brain-stem center is highly implicated in acute panic experience, the *raphe nucleus*. This nucleus is located near the LC and it is known that they affect each other, though the raphe nucleus uses a different chemical transmitter called *serotonin*. Drugs that block the action of either nor-epinephrine or serotonin are effective in stopping many panic attacks. Although it is not yet known precisely how these structures generate panic, it is clear now that they are intimately involved in the most basic physical symptoms of a panic attack. These areas of the brain stem are also connected to higher brain centers in the *limbic system* that underlie our broader emotional responding.

The Anticipatory Anxiety

The *limbic system* is the area of the brain that has been implicated in anticipatory anxiety. This is a broad area, with a number of specific structures located in the central core of the brain. The limbic system has long been known to be central to many emotional responses, including anger and fear. Jeffrey Gray, a British psychologist, has demonstrated that the LC and the *hippocampus*, a structure in the limbic system, interact to produce anticipatory anxiety.[32] It is further known that the hippocampus as well as other parts of the limbic system are highly responsive to a class of tranquilizing drugs called the *benzodiazepines*, of which Valium and Xanax are examples (see Chapter 10). This hippocampal area is thought to be affected by LC-related panic and, in turn, the hippocampus is sensitized by these effects so that its continued activity is experienced as *anticipatory anxiety*, or fear of having another panic. In turn, Gorman and colleagues postulated that continued anticipation of having an attack may indeed lead to a full panic by the stimulation of LC and other brain-stem structures by the limbic system's anticipatory anxiety.

This theoretical picture of how activation of brain structures relates to anticipatory anxiety and to panic also helps explain how various treatments work. Antipanic drugs seem to raise the firing threshold of LC neurons; that is, they make them less excitable so that even if the limbic system is sending messages of anticipatory anxiety, it is not enough to make the LC fire into a panic attack. Psychological treatment techniques like relaxation training and breathing retraining (described in Chapter 8) that lower activity in the limbic area seem to work by decreasing the limbic area's signals to the LC, thus keeping it from firing in a panic attack.

Phobic Avoidance

The third central component of panic disorder and agoraphobia is the feature of strong avoidance of places where the person believes that he or she might have another attack. The area of the brain believed to support this behavior is the *prefrontal cortex*. This area is one of the most highly evolved areas of the brain and one which clearly sets humans above the lower animals. This is an area in which our higher mental processes take place, such as the ability to see many relationships among objects and situations. The prefrontal cortex is where we are able to form connections between the symptoms we experience, the situation in which we experience them, our labeling of those situations as "dangerous," and all the associated thoughts we might have had about them. Most likely this human capacity maintains the intense avoidance we call agoraphobia that we see following an attack of panic. When humans experience a panic attack, their higher mental abilities allow their imaginations to conceive of many terrible things that might be happening to them. Their ability to think of other places where it "might" occur again logically leads them to avoid such places. Who would reenter a situation in which you have experienced the most horrifying experience of your life?

Anatomically, this prefrontal cortex lies at some distance from the brain stem and limbic areas that are involved in other aspects of the panic. However, clear neural pathways connect these areas so that they can be in close communication. Treatment for the avoidance component of panic-agoraphobia must then focus on changing these learned beliefs and bringing the person to the point that he or she can reenter situations in which attacks have occurred without allowing another one to occur; that is, unlearning the fear and avoidance responses. (Techniques for achieving this relearning will be described in Chapters 8 and 9.) This neuroanatomical theory proposed by Gorman and his colleagues is of value because it integrates knowledge of neuroanatomy, psychiatry, and psychology. Furthermore, it is generally compatible with the next theoretical approach which details more of the psychological processes involved in the initiation and maintenance of panic anxiety and agoraphobic avoidance.

A Biopsychosocial Theory of Panic and Agoraphobia

David Barlow's theory concerning the origins and nature of panic disorder and agoraphobia seems to take off where Gorman's theory leaves off. Barlow's conception focuses more on the psychological aspects of how the person is affected by his or her environment and how this reaction leads to panic and agoraphobia. To begin, Barlow accepts the well-documented findings that indicate there is a biological contribution to panic that is most likely hereditary. Clearly, panic is more likely to appear in other members of a family if one member has panic disorder. Further, Torgersen's data from the twin studies show that anxiety disorders have a hereditary component to them, even though it is not at all clear at this point just what is inherited. It does not appear to be specific behavior patterns associated with panic or agoraphobia. Barlow, like others, believes that what is inherited is a *vulnerability* to develop anxiety disorders. The specific vulnerability is an overly reactive autonomic nervous system. This highly responsive ANS is controlled by the brain centers outlined in Gorman's theory.

The second element of Barlow's theory concerns the effects of life stresses. A number of research studies of people with panic disorder and recurrent panic attacks have demonstrated that panickers experienced significant negative life events that are seen as stressors, coincident in time with the onset of the first panic. These stressors tend to be of interpersonal loss, death of a loved one, divorce, birth of a child, major surgery, and school or work stresses. Experienced by those who are biologically vulnerable to high ANS reactivity, these stresses can lead to the first panic attack. Other factors may enter here as well that affect the outcome of these stresses. There is good evidence now that persons who feel that they have the psychological support of important others in their lives are less affected by major stresses. Those who feel alone and without social support are more vulnerable to stress effects. This analysis of panics fits well some recent data collected on adolescents by Jennifer Lee Macaulay and myself, which I mentioned previously. We found that reported stressors, especially from school and family, were highly associated with the more severe panic experiences. Low social support, especially from family, was also highly related to severity of panic attacks, just as predicted by Barlow's theory. The following case example clearly illustrates how these factors can culminate in a series of panics.

> Gertrude was a 34-year-old mother of five children. She had always characterized herself as one who could remain calm and cope with any crisis situation. She felt she was just not the type to panic. However, shortly after her sixth child was born, Gertrude was stricken with what turned out to be a panic attack. Thinking it was a heart attack or some such catastrophe, she had her husband drive her to the hospital emergency room where she was told it was just nerves. An additional element that seems to have contributed to the onset of this panic was that at this same time her husband had taken a new job which would require him to be gone from home more than he had in the past. Shortly thereafter, she was stricken with a second attack. Again, she went to the emergency room where again she was told it was just nerves. By the time of the third attack, she was too embarrassed to go into the emergency room so she had her husband drive her around the hospital so they would be close to the ER in case they needed to go in. This time the attack subsided without her going into the ER. She came to believe that it was just

stress and her husband's response had shown her that he would not abandon her. With this realization and his show of support, she never had another attack.

Panic attacks like Gertrude's are called "false alarms" in Barlow's theory. They are full-fledged fight-or-flight alarm responses, even though the threat to which they are reacting is somewhat remote. The mobilization of energy does not help the person escape from an imminent danger; there is no physical threat. Thus, they are false alarms. At the time, the victims may not make the connection between the panic and the stresses they are experiencing since they are typically not occurring at that moment. The attack therefore seems to come out of the blue and to be unrelated to anything external.

Following such false alarms, some people seem to shrug them off whereas others go on to become fully consumed by them as panic disordered or agoraphobic. Recall that as many as 36 percent of some adult samples have reported such attacks. Few became panic disordered. Several factors may be important in determining what happens next. For some people, a strong association is made between the frightening attack itself and the situation in which it occurred. If an attack hits while a person is driving, later even thinking about driving may bring on an anxiety reaction recalling the panic. The person may then anticipate that if he drives again, another attack may occur. This keeps the fear of the attack alive, and the many environmental cues associated with driving can maintain the anxiety. At this point, panic attacks, elicited by associated stimuli, including thoughts that have become associated with the false alarm, can be called *learned alarms*—learned through association. This association is a version of classical or Pavlovian conditioning.

It is also possible that internal bodily signs associated with the false alarm attack can become learned cues to recall the experience and elicit learned alarms. If dizziness were one prominent symptom experienced during the false alarm, later occurrences of dizziness, as the result of standing up too quickly, may recall the whole attack and actually elicit part or all of the panic symptoms. This was the situation with Sally.

During most of Sally's numerous panics, she typically experienced dizziness. One day, while lying on the floor to relax a strained neck muscle, she was called by her children. Without thinking, she got up too quickly, causing a momentary dizziness. Since dizziness had so often been associated with her panic attacks, it now automatically elicited a full and intense panic attack that lasted for hours. This effect occurred even though she rationally knew that her dizziness was only due to rising too quickly after having been relaxing.

Internal bodily changes from a variety of activities are capable of eliciting panics in a way similar to those of Sally. For example, exercise, climbing a flight of stairs, or getting up abruptly can all cause an immediate increase in heart rate and therefore are capable of eliciting panics in those so prone. Heart-rate changes associated with sleep cycles as well may explain unexpected panics elicited while sound asleep. Thus, normal bodily changes or sensations, through association with panics, can quite innocently become cues for setting off a panic attack, just as cues from the external environment can elicit attacks. This may also be the basis of relaxation-induced anxiety mentioned previously.

In addition to the learning or conditioning mechanisms, several other psychological factors appear to be related to increasing the chances that a person will have continuing panic attacks. Those persons who are prone to worry about what happened and who continue to worry about the possibilities of having more attacks may be maintained in a relatively constant state of anticipatory anxiety. Barlow calls this "anxious apprehension." One who is anxiously on the alert for signs that another attack may occur would be in a constant state of arousal that could actually make it more likely that they would indeed have another attack. This could be particularly true if the individual was hyperattentive to all bodily changes and was prone to mis-interpret normal bodily sensations as signs of impending panic symptoms.

This cognitive misinterpretation, often seen in panic and agoraphobic persons, has become the center of some theoretical accounts of the onset and maintenence of these conditions.[33]

The apprehensively anxious person who continually scans his or her body for signs that an anxiety attack may be in the offing is bound to find something to focus on. This bodily focus and consequent anxiety can then escalate into an actual panic attack. The following case illustrates how such misinterpretation of bodily signs can be panic eliciting and how correction of these misinterpretations can be therapeutic.

> Sara had a long history of panic and agoraphobia but was making progress in therapy to the point that she felt she could venture out to a restaurant with her husband. While awaiting the arrival of their dinner, Sara was somewhat apprehensive about the possibility of having a panic attack. Her general anxiety over her possibly having an attack was accentuated by the fussing of a family with small children at a nearby table. The milk spilling, food throwing, and children whining accumulated to upset her to the point that she was beginning to experience the onset of a panic attack. She was just about to escape from the restaurant as she could tolerate the anxiety no longer, when she realized something that had been discussed in therapy; that when she experienced these signs, she should be sure that she was not misinterpreting just any signs of arousal as panic. As she reevaluated her feelings, she realized that what she was feeling was anger at the family for disrupting her din-ner. As she more accurately labeled her emotional state as anger, the sense of rising panic diminished and she no longer felt the need to escape. After the family left, she and her husband were able to enjoy the remainder of their dinner.

An additional psychological factor that surely contributes to increased chances of having recurrent panic attacks is a sense that one has no control over what is happening. This sense of not having control over one's reaction is probably the most frightening aspect of panic and is at least part of the reason people maintain their agoraphobic avoidance. If you do not believe you have control over your reaction, then you might have an attack anytime and there is nothing that you can do about it. You are literally at the mercy of whatever is causing them. The effect on panic of this belief concerning lack of control was convincingly illustrated in a recent study by Barlow's research team.[34] These researchers enlisted a group of patients with panic disorder to participate in an experiment in which they were to inhale a solution of oxygen and carbon dioxide. Inhalation of this particular mixture has been shown to elicit panic attacks in most panic-disordered patients. This experimental induction of panic has become one of the ways that panic disorder can be studied under laboratory conditions. In this experiment, the researchers' task was to create in some patients an illusion of control over their panic symptoms while not giving that illusion of control to others. The researchers could then examine whether and to what extent the illusion influenced the panic. After all patients had been fully informed of what they might experience during the experiment and they signed appropriate voluntary consent forms, they were taken individually into a booth in which they would inhale the gas mixture. They were told that, during the inhalation, a light might come on in the booth, and if it did, it meant that they could control with a dial the amount of oxygen and carbon dioxide they were inhaling and thereby control any panic symptoms they were feeling. The light was programmed to come on randomly for half of the patients but not for the other half. In fact, however, even if the light came on, the dial was not connected to the inhalation apparatus and thus afforded no real control for the patients in any way. The only real differences between the two groups was that with the light coming on, the one group was led to "believe" they had control while the other was not.

The effect of this belief or its absence on the patients' panic experience was dramatic. Significantly more of the patients in the "no light, no illusion" group experienced full clinical-level panic attacks. The symptoms this group experienced were more intense and they reported their experience more similar to attacks they typically experienced in their everyday environments, compared with the "illusion of control" group. These researchers hypothesized that the gas inhalation causes unpleasant feelings to which many panic-disordered people may be particularly sensitive. When these feelings are perceived as signs of an impending uncontrollable panic attack, they can cause the patient's anxiety to escalate into a full-blown panic attack. Additionally, these changes in bodily sensations elicited by the inhalation may, through their association with previous attacks, come to elicit the full panic syndrome. This relationship was noted in the case of Sally, whose dizziness from getting up too abruptly precipitated her attack.

The effect of experiencing sensations that either trigger automatic panic or thoughts that a panic might ensue may happen from any number of relatively common everyday experiences. For example, hyperventilation—rapid shallow breathing—produces physical sensations similar to those of the inhalation in this study. Some theorists believe that much panic disorder is a result of symptoms produced by hyperventilation which frighten the person and, in turn, escalates into full panics.[35]

SUMMARY AND CONCLUSIONS

Panic disorder and its common result agoraphobic avoidance of numerous situations can virtually paralyze those who are afflicted. We know that panic attacks have plagued humans for thousands, perhaps millions of years, since the ancient Greeks blamed the disorder on the fun-loving god Pan. The sudden, inexplicable terror that overtakes a person is apparently experienced by as many as one third of all adults. Fortunately, only one to three percent of adults experience them with sufficient frequency that they can be called panic disorder. However, it is becoming increasingly evident that adolescents and even young children experience these terrors. These attacks, like all human experiences, must be generated at some level of our brains. Research and theory today seem to be integrating the knowledge of the working of the brain with the effects of psychological and environmental stressors in such a way that all these elements can now be seen to figure in when explaining the occurrence of panics. As will be illustrated in Chapters 8, 9, and 10, these advances have also been translated into highly effective treatment techniques. Although the panic disordered and agoraphobic patient can be virtually immobilized and housebound, there are current treatment methods that can reach out to them and provide them with relief of their fear and suffering.

REFERENCES

1. Judy Mills, "The Beast Within: The Dark Side of the Mind/Body Connection," *Washington* (Jan/Feb, 1989), 65.
2. G. Ron Norton, B. Harrison, J. Hauch, and L. Rhodes, "Characteristics of People with Infrequent Panic Attacks," *Journal of Abnormal Psychology* 94 (1985): 216–221.
3. Jennifer Lee Macaulay and Ronald Kleinknecht, "Panic and Panic Attacks in Adolescents," *Journal of Anxiety Disorders* 3 (1989): 221–241.
4. Timothy Brown and Thomas Cash, "The Phenomenon of Nonclinical Panic: Panic, Fear, and Avoidance," *Journal of Anxiety Disorders* 4 (1990): 15–30.
5. Michael Von Korff, W. Eaton, and P. Keyl, "The Epidemiology of Panic Attacks and Panic Disorder," *American Journal of Epidemiology* 122 (1985): 970–981.
6. Hans-Ulrich Wittchen, "Natural Course and Spontaneous Remissions of Untreated Anxiety Disorders: Results of the Munich Follow-up Study (MFS)," in *Panic and Phobias II: Treatments and Variables Affecting Course and Outcome,* Iver Hand and Hans-Ulrich Wittchen, ed. (New York: Springer-Verlag, 1988).
7. Ronald Rapee, J. Ancis, and David Barlow, "Emotional Reactions to Physiological Sensations: Comparison of Panic Disorder and Non-clinical Subjects," *Behaviour Research and therapy* 25 (1987): 265–270.
8. Donald Klein and Hilary Klein, "The Substantive Effect of Variations in Panic Measurement and Agoraphobia," *Journal of Anxiety Disorders* 3 (1989): 45–56.

9. Paul Lelliott and Isaac Marks, "Onset of Panic Disorder with Agoraphobia," *Archives of General Psychiatry* 46 (1990): 1000–1104.

10. Jennifer Lee Macaulay and Ronald Kleinknecht, "Panic and Panic Attacks in Adolescents," *Journal of Anxiety Disorders* 3 (1989): 221–241.

11. Janet Klosko, Robert Rotunda, and David Barlow, "A Descriptive Study of First Panic Attacks of Patients Diagnosed with Agoraphobia with Panic Attacks or Panic Disorder." Paper presented to the Annual Meeting of the Association for the Advancement of Behavior Therapy, Chicago (Nov. 1986).

12. Allan Cohen, David Barlow, and Edward Blanchard, "The Psychophysiology of Relaxation Associated Panic Attacks," *Journal of Abnormal Psychology* 94 (1985): 96–101.

13. Jerome Myers, Myrna Weissman, Gary Tischler, Charles Holzer, III, Philip Leaf, Helen Orvaschel, James Anthony, Jeffrey Boyd, Jack Burke, Morton Kramer, and Roger Stoltzman, "Six Month Prevalence of Psychiatric Disorders in Three Communities," *Archives of General Psychiatry* 41 (1984): 959–967.

14. Ibid.

15. Von Korff, Eaton, and Keyl, "The Epidemiology of Panic Attacks," 970–981.

16. Donna Moreau, Myrna Weissman, and V. Warner, "Panic Disorder in Children: Six Case Reports." Paper presented to the Annual Meeting of the American Psychiatric Association, Montreal, Canada (May, 1988).

17. Raymond Crowe, Russell Noyes, D. L. Pauls, and D. Slymen, "A Family Study of Panic Disorder," *Archives of General Psychiatry* 40 (1983): 1065–1069.

18. Svenn Torgersen, "Genetic Factors in Anxiety Disorders," *Archives of General Psychiatry* 40 (1983): 1085–1089.

19. David Barlow and Jerome Cerny, *Psychological Treatment of Panic* (New York: Guilford Press, 1988).

20. Alan Goldstein and Diane Chambless, "A Reanalysis of Agoraphobia," *Behavior Therapy* 9 (1978): 47–59.

21. R. S. Hallam and R. G. Hafner, "Fears of Phobic Patients: Factor Analysis of Self-Report Data," *Behaviour Research and Therapy* 16 (1978): 1–6.

22. David Barlow, Peter DiNardo, B. Vermilyea, J. A. Vermilyea, and Edward Blanchard, "Co-Morbidity among Anxiety Disorders: Issues in Diagnosis and Classification," *Journal of Nervous and Mental Disease* 1174 (1986): 63–72.

23. Myrna Weismann, Gerald Klerman, Jeffrey Markowitz, and Robert Ouellette, "Suicidal Ideation and Suicide Attempts in Panic Disorder and Attacks," *New England Journal of Medicine* 321 (1989): 1209–1214.

24. Matt Kushner, Kenneth Sher, and Bernard Beitman, "The Relation between Alcohol Problems and the Anxiety Disorders," *American Journal of Psychiatry* 147 (1990): 685–995.

25. Ibid.

26. David Barlow, *Anxiety and Its Disorders* (New York: Guilford Press, 1988).

27. Lelliott and Marks, "Onset of Panic Disorder," 1000–1104.

28. Barlow, *Anxiety and Its Disorders.*

29. David Sheehan, *The Anxiety Disease* (New York: Scribner and Sons, 1983).
30. Jack Gorman, Michael Liebowitz, Abby Fryer, and Jonathan Stein, "A Neuroanatomical Hypothesis for Panic Disorder," *American Journal of Psychiatry* 146 (1989): 148–161.
31. Barlow, *Anxiety and its Disorders*.
32. Jeffrey Gray, *Psychology of Fear and Stress*, 2nd ed. (Cambridge, England: Cambridge University Press, 1987).
33. David Clark, "A Cognitive Approach to Panic," *Behaviour Research and Therapy* 24 (1986): 461–470.
34. William Sanderson, David Barlow, and Ronald Rapee, "The Influence of an Illusion of Control on Panic Attacks Induced via Inhalation of 5.5% Carbon Dioxide-Enriched Air," *Archives of General Psychiatry* 46 (1988): 157–162.
35. Ronald Ley, "Agoraphobia, The Panic Attack and Hyperventilation Syndrome," *Behaviour Research and Therapy* 23 (1985): 79–81.

Posttraumatic Stress, Generalized Anxiety, and Obsessive-Compulsive Disorders

POSTTRAUMATIC STRESS DISORDER

We have all heard the comment in reference to a person who has just endured a severe trauma that he or she "will be scarred for life" and, indeed, there are traumas that do scar people and, in some cases, for the rest of their lives. Awareness that trauma can be indelibly printed in a person's mind and affect his or her behavior has long been known. Robert Burton (1577–1640), the English clergyman, scholar, and author, described in some detail a case history that today might be diagnosed as posttraumatic stress disorder.[1] In describing the psychological aftermath of an earthquake, Burton reported that

> whole streets and . . . palaces were overturned . . . , there was such a hideous noise, . . . like thunder, and filthy smell, . . . their hearts quaked, and men and beasts were incredibly terrified.[2]

In describing the effects on people he wrote:

> Many were bereft of their senses; and others . . . knew not
> what they did. Balsius . . . was so affrighted for his part,
> that though it were two months after, he was scarcely his
> own man, neither could he drive the remembrance of it out
> of his mind. . . . some years following, they will tremble
> afresh at the remembrance . . . even all their lives long, if
> mention is made of it.[3]

The human reaction to disasters and traumas, both natural and man-made that Burton so aptly captured has most likely been with us for as long as we have been human, and possibly before that. Other terms have been used to describe this emotional and behavioral pattern of reaction to trauma. Wars, of course, produce many such cases variously called *shell shock* or *combat fatigue*. Effects on survivors of human-inflicted atrocities have been referred to as *survivors' syndrome*. Rape victims who experience such violation have been said to suffer from *rape trauma syndrome*. All share a common pattern of emotional reactions. All these terms have now come under the common heading of posttraumatic stress disorder (PTSD).

Symptoms of PTSD

One of the prominent symptoms of PTSD is that after experiencing a trauma that is beyond the range of normal human experience, the person acts or feels as if he or she were reexperiencing the trauma. This reexperiencing of the trauma may occur as intrusive memories and dreams that are especially apt to occur on the anniversaries of the trauma and when exposed to situations that call the event to mind again.

Also a part of the reaction is that the person suffering PTSD would attempt to avoid situations or thoughts that might rekindle memories of the traumas. In some cases, they might demonstrate amnesia for the event, show a decreased interest in activities and people they previously enjoyed, and find that they are unable to feel as deeply as they used to. Some report a sense that they have no future ahead of them.

Physical symptoms and mood changes are common as well, including sleep difficulties, irritable or angry moods, high reactivity (startle) to sudden noises, and difficulty concentrating. For some sufferers, the symptoms are delayed and do not develop for months or years following the traumatic event. James Nicholson and, to a lesser extent, his wife Cynthia, experienced many of these symptoms for over a year following what began as a pleasant birthday dinner with friends at a local restaurant.

> While lingering over an after-dinner drink, the party was not aware that it had neared closing time. Although the group had apparently not heard, the bartender had asked them to leave so he could close. The next thing James recalled, he was being helped up off the floor, groggy and confused. Seemingly unprovoked, the burly bartender had hit James full force along the side of his head, knocking him to the floor and rendering James partially unconscious. As the party gathered their coats and the birthday presents and moved outside, the bartender followed and again attacked James from the rear, this time knocking him totally unconscious. His friends got him away, revived him, and then had to restrain James from going back to look for the bartender. Badly shaken, they took James home.
>
> James's responses from that point on until he sought treatment were textbook signs of PTSD. Although a large and husky person, James had always been a quiet, mild, and sensitive person who had never been in a fight himself. Now he was constantly angry, on edge, and unable to control his emotions. He felt "pumped up with adrenaline" all the time. He became upset with himself for not being able to calm down and lost confidence in his work and in his ability to make decisions. He became highly reactive to any sign of argument or disagreement by others. This seemed to rekindle his full emotional reaction to

the assault. A sudden move or sharp sound would startle him, sending him into a panic. He smashed a small mouse he found in the yard, another previously uncharacteristic behavior. James experienced insomnia, nightmares concerning the fight, and was plagued by gastrointestinal upset. He and the whole family were upset by his reactions. By the time they appeared for therapy a year later, they had not gone out with friends, because James was afraid to be alone away from home, and Cynthia had developed insomnia and back problems. The children were often frightened and refused to go to school, apparently knowing that something was wrong at home. As legal action was pending and they had to describe the incident repeatedly and in great detail, the intensity of James's distress and the disruption in the family increased to where it became intolerable.

Who Gets PTSD?

Many of the symptoms experienced by James were also described by Burton some 370 years ago. They could not get the traumas out of their minds, they were plagued for all their lives and were scarcely themselves. Exactly how many people experience PTSD is difficult to say as prevalence figures from various sources are quite divergent. Figures from the large surveys that supplied prevalence rates for other disorders are less clear here, but for St. Louis, Missouri, 0.5 percent of males and 1.3 percent of females were found to meet the criteria for PTSD diagnosis.[4] In these cases, most of the males so diagnosed were Viet Nam veterans and most of the females had been victims of sexual assault.

Most of our reliable knowledge of PTSD has been obtained in recent years, largely from two groups of individuals: veterans of the Viet Nam war and victims of sexual assault. Overall, 14.7 percent of Viet Nam veterans at some time had PTSD.[5] Among those who saw action but were not wounded, only 3 percent were affected, whereas among the wounded, 20 percent had PTSD.

In a recent study aimed at obtaining more reliable information concerning crime-related effects on women, Dean Kilpatrick and his colleagues at the Medical University of South Carolina in Charleston conducted a large-scale investigation.[6] They found that of a representative sample of Charleston women, over 75 percent had been crime victims. Of these, 27.8 percent either were currently or had at some point suffered PTSD from their crime experience. Among those whose victimization had been a completed rape, 57.1 percent had PTSD. Thus, some investigators like Kilpatrick suggest that the prevalence of PTSD is considerably higher than previously thought. He believes that 6 percent of adult women currently experience crime-related PTSD alone.

Although it appears that a large percentage of victims of severe trauma as war and sexual assault experience post-traumatic stress, it is also apparent that many people do not develop the disorders. S. J. Rachman of the University of British Columbia has focused on the reverse side; that is, those who are exposed to extraordinary trauma and do not show signs of anxiety.[7] Even the great majority of wounded war veterans did not develop PTSD. Rachman points to the bombing of England during World War II and of Japan, where massive damage was done; yet symptoms of PTSD were relatively rare among the victims. What then are the factors that determine who becomes distressed and who does not?

Although all the factors that determine who does and who does not develop PTSD are not yet clear, several have been identified that are clearly involved in most cases. Probably the single most important factor determining who develops the disorder is the severity and intensity of exposure to the stressor. Those who have been exposed most directly and intensely are most likely to develop the symptoms. In war situations, those soldiers who saw the most direct and intense combat were more likely to develop symptoms. And among those who saw intense combat, those who were wounded were more likely to develop PTSD than those who were not wounded.[8]

Intensity of exposure to the stressor is also most predictive of who among rape victims develops PTSD. Dean Kilpatrick and his colleagues in Charleston found that three factors were highly related to symptom development: (1) whether the rape was completed, (2) whether physical injury resulted, and (3) whether the victim perceived herself as being in mortal danger.[9] The woman who was injured during a completed rape and who believed she was going to be killed was most likely to develop PTSD symptoms.

Although less strongly predictive of symptom formation was the finding by researchers among war veterans that those who had a family history of mental disorder, who had a prior or current history of mental disorder, or who had been involved in drug abuse also were more likely to experience PTSD symptoms. These factors were mainly predictive of PTSD among those with less direct and intense combat experience. If the war experience itself was severe enough, this was a strong enough factor that it would override any other possible risk factors. Among those with very intense combat experiences, factors such as family history were irrelevant in their development of PTSD.

Among rape victims, an additional factor may be related to symptom development. If the rape occurred in a place that the person believed to be safe, the chances are greater that PTSD will occur. If the woman had believed some particular place was safe but has now been shown that there is no such place, she has reason to fear all places, including those that had been unsafe before as well as those that were once considered safe. If one were led to believe that there are no refuges from danger, one would become wary, reactive, and always on edge.

Finally, another factor related to development or lack of development of symptoms is the degree of social support the person has from others. Those victims who believe they can rely on a network of friends and/or family to help them through the immediate aftermath of the trauma are less likely to develop symptoms than those who perceive themselves to be alone. This factor of social support is a buffer against the many negative effects of all kinds of stress. Of course, this could be one of the reasons why those involved in the World War II bombings of their homelands were less likely than military forces in combat to develop stress-related symptoms. Having your own people and being in familiar surroundings are sources of comfort.

A Cognitive Theory of PTSD

Edna Foa and Michael Kozak proposed a theory of the development of PTSD that seems to help us understand some of the facts that are known.[10] They proposed that the traumatic experience and all the stimuli and responses associated with it become firmly linked together in a memory structure in the brain. This memory structure is like a network of mental representations of the traumatic incident. It is analogous to a computer program that, once stimulated to run, goes through a series of operations. The purpose of the program and its operations is to enable the person to escape danger. When any element of this memory structure is stimulated or accessed, its connections with other elements in the network bring them on-line and the system of escape responses initially elicited at the trauma is again activated. The person then reacts physically, behaviorally, and emotionally, just as was done at the original event while this memory structure runs through its program.

While we have many such memory networks in our brains that link together the various elements of our world, "fear networks" differ in that they contain the meaning of situations with respect to danger. Since many elements may be associated with one another, so that we remember things that are related through their networks, when these networks contain danger information, they become fear networks. Fear networks, when accessed, set off the escape behavior and reactivate the original experience. Stimulation of such networks would seem to explain why PTSD victims frequently report that certain stimuli, those that access the fear network, vividly reactivate the whole experience in the form of a flashback. A car backfiring can send a veteran with PTSD diving for cover; an inadvertent touch on the shoulder can trigger an hysterical panic episode in a PTSD rape victim. Unless this strong element of danger is involved, the network is only a regular memory structure. An example of how information can change this more normal memory structure to a fear structure is well illustrated in a case reported by Dean Kilpatrick, which was noted by Foa and her colleagues. Following a traumatic rape, a woman, although understandably shaken, had not developed the symptoms of PTSD as might be expected. It was only several months later, after she learned that her rapist had killed his next victim, that she developed PTSD symptoms. It was as though when she fully realized the serious danger that she had been in, the memory structure became a fear network that elicited the symptoms and escape program. Thus, the information that she had been in mortal danger was added to the memory network and transformed it into a highly reactive fear program that now included the reactivation of the traumatic experience and the associated escape responses.

This theory of fear networks is similar in many ways to the theory of panic disorder proposed by David Barlow.[11] In his theory, certain elements of the original response, when later experienced, for various reasons, could activate the full panic episode as if it were a "panic program."

GENERALIZED ANXIETY DISORDER

The person with generalized anxiety disorder (GAD) is a chronic worrier and most likely has been for some years. To the person with GAD, many things are potential disasters waiting to happen. In one sample of GAD patients collected by Barlow and his colleagues, 100 percent of them endorsed the statement that they "worried excessively about minor things."[12]

Defining Symptoms

The major defining characteristic of GAD diagnosis is excessive worry about possible life circumstances and misfortunes. However, people with this disorder are not particularly different from most other people in that the issues they worry about are family, money, work, and illness. Not only do they profess to worry most of the time, they also exhibit numerous anxiety-related symptoms: *motor tension* (jumpiness, jitteriness, and muscle tension); *ANS hyperactivity* (sweating, rapid heartbeat, cold clammy hands, feeling of a lump in the throat); *vigilance and scanning* (hyperattentiveness). These symptoms, in turn, result in the person's being easily distracted, unable to concentrate, irritable, and unable to sleep.[13]

Generalized anxiety disorder is relatively new as a formal category of mental disorder and thus its full characteristics and defining boundaries have not yet been fully clarified.[14] While many people are prone to worry, all worriers should not be diagnosed as GAD. The major difference between GAD and "normal" worry is that the person with GAD worries more constantly, and the worries tend to be more unrealistic. This constant level of anxiety keeps the person on edge most of the time, although it typically causes only mild social or economic impairment.

Although people with GAD may experience occasional surges of high anxiety and even panic attacks in many cases, it is their mostly constant state of worry, tension, and arousal that differentiates them from those suffering the other anxiety disorders. Further, even though many people receiving other anxiety diagnoses also qualify for GAD, the generalized anxiety appears to be at least partially separate from the other disorders. Some have found that for those with additional anxiety disorder diagnoses, for example, panic disorder, when the panic is treated, the generalized anxiety remains and necessitates separate treatment programs.

Prevalence and Onset

Considerable debate exists over the true population prevalence of people who worry and react with sufficient intensity to qualify for the diagnosis of GAD. Most current estimates of the population prevalence of GAD range from 2.5 percent[15] to 6.4 percent.[16] Like the other anxiety disorders, GAD shows a two-thirds majority of females, although some clinical samples have not found this discrepancy.[17]

GAD appears to have a more gradual and earlier onset then PD. Anderson and her colleagues report a mean onset at about 16 years of age, nearly 7 years earlier than for their subjects with panic disorder.[18] Thus, it also appears to be more chronic in its course, having been with the person for many years by the time they seek treatment. Many readily express the fact that they have been worriers all their lives and cannot point to a date of onset.

> Margaret, who was 60 years of age, recently sought treatment at the request of her physician and at the insistence of her husband. She was increasingly reluctant to travel to visit friends and family and had come to need "nerve pills" to allow her to travel to visit her grown children who lived in other parts of the country. Her worry over travel had progressed to the point at which she would much rather stay home than travel, even to visit her grandchildren. Although travel in any form was a problem for her, her fear was not simply a phobia of driving, flying, or travel in general, nor was it the only worry she exhibited. Her concern with travel was composed of a variety of related excessive worries. She worried days in advance before they left and never slept the night before a trip. On the freeways she worried about every car within sight; in cities she worried about getting lost; on mountain passes, she worried about the car breaking down, being stranded; and she was always concerned about running out of money.
>
> Margaret had felt this worry as long as she could remember, even as a child. It had escalated in the past few years when some of her fears associated with traveling were realized: she fell asleep in the car and they had an accident. Later, the car engine burned up while they were 2,000 miles away from home and it had cost them $5,000. These incidents only solidified her already well-developed

belief system that if things could go wrong, they would go wrong.

Although many people like Margaret with GAD seem to have always been chronic worriers, other evidence suggests that the experience of certain life events can be associated with the onset of GAD.[19] In a recent epidemiological study that sampled over 2,000 individuals, it was found that men who reported experiencing four or more significant life events during the preceding 12 months had 8.5 times the risk of developing GAD when evaluated. The association between numerous life events and GAD onset was not present for women in this study. Furthermore, in contrast to panic disorder, GAD seems to have little or no familial and/or genetic component.[20,21]

OBSESSIVE-COMPULSIVE DISORDER

The category of obsessive-compulsive disorder has two related components: obsessions that are recurrent thoughts, ideas, or images, and compulsions that are stereotypic, repetitive acts. As with common fears, most of us experience mild versions of these obsessions, like the tune or radio commercial that we cannot seem to get out of our mind or the thought that perhaps we forgot to turn the water off in the bathroom. However, for the person with obsessive-compulsive disorder, the thoughts or actions do not go away so readily. In its more extreme forms, it becomes the most disabling and immobilizing of all the anxiety disorders.

Obsessions

In contrast to the recurring tunes or jingles that we may experience as nuisances, obsessions typically have a disturbing, morbid, or frightening quality to them. Another defining characteristic of clinical obsessions is that they appear to be largely out of the person's volitional control. It is as if they are being forced upon the person's consciousness and are therefore seen as alien or foreign to the person's personality. To describe this intrusive quality of obsessions, the term *ego-alien* is often used.[22] The person attempts to ignore or suppress the obsessions but such attempts are typically unsuccessful, at least in the long run. The resulting sense of lack of control may be as anxiety provoking and disturbing as the content of the obsessions.

The Content of the Obsessions

The most common themes of obsessions involve dirt and contamination. These obsessions, reported by up to 46 percent of one group of obsessive-compulsive patients, center on thoughts and fears that they would develop some disease if they came into contact with virtually any object.[23] Obsessions can become quite debilitating, since one of the major sources feared is door knobs. For example, one patient had an obsession with contamination and could not open a door with her bare hand. She would carry gloves or a clean cloth to drape over objects she needed to touch in order to prevent direct contact with any object. She could not shake bare hands with another person. This particular obsession is typically associated with compulsive cleaning rituals as well. In fact, between 70 and 80 percent of persons with obsessions also have compulsions.[24-26]

The second common theme of obsessions involves thoughts or images concerning aggression or harm. Approximately one quarter of obsessional patients report themes often involving harm or injury to loved ones. Behaviorally, this harm obsession results in the individual's constantly worrying about others and checking on their safety or performing rituals to ensure their safety.

Concern with orderliness is also a common theme reported by somewhere between 23 percent and 35 percent of patients.[27,28] Approximately half of those patients with obsessions report more than a single theme.[29]

The Form of Obsessions

In addition to the different contents of obsessions, they also take different forms. An investigation by Akhter and his colleagues revealed five different forms of obsessions.[30] As with the different content themes, any individual may have more than one form of obsession. *Obsessive doubts* were the most frequent, being reported by 75 percent of the sample. These doubts were characterized by the individual who persistently worried that some task had not been satisfactorily completed. Examples include doubts that a door had been locked, a window closed, or water turned off. These doubts continued to intrude into the person's awareness, even though the person rationally knew that, in fact, it had been taken care of.

Obsessive thoughts were described by 34 percent of patients as seemingly uncontrolled endless trains of thoughts. These thoughts typically concerned long scenarios of events that might occur in the future, or that germs were everywhere, and what would happen if the person were to become contaminated.

Obsessive impulses, described by 17 percent of the patients, involved powerful urges to perform certain acts that would seem silly and embarrassing or that involved assaultive acts toward others. Common obsessive impulses that were described included, "I feel I will shout obscenities in the street," "I'm afraid that if I am around sharp objects, like knives, I will harm someone." As described by Akhter, a lawyer from India had an urge to drink from his inkpot.[31] Although this is a rather silly and mild obsession, the lawyer also felt frightening urges to strangle his son. Fortunately, such urges, although bothersome and even frightening, are probably never actually carried out.

Obsessive fears, noted by 36 percent of Akhter's group, involved fear of losing control of oneself and perhaps doing embarrassing things. For example, a school teacher feared that he would tell his class about his unsatisfactory sexual relations with his wife. Of course he did not want to do this, nor did he have an urge to do so. But he feared that he might.

Obsessional images, reported by 7 percent of the group, involve scenes of mutilated bodies, a loved one having a serious accident, or someone being violently assaulted. Akhter described one patient who on entering her bathroom experienced an image of her baby being flushed down the toilet.[32]

Such scenes, impulses, and fears of embarrassment keep the person in a constant state of anxiety. And as noted previously, a majority of persons who experience obsessions also engage in compulsive acts that are related to their obsessions.

Compulsions

In the same way that obsessions are intrusions into a person's mental or cognitive activity, compulsions are intrusions into his or her behavior. Compulsions are repetitive behaviors or acts that a person feels compelled to perform. Often these acts, which are conducted in a stereotypic and mechanical fashion, are usually recognized by the person as being excessive and senseless. Although there may be a semblance of volitional control over the actions under some conditions, the urge is so strongly experienced that, in practice, control is quite minimal.[33] At least during the early phase of the disorder, the person also has a desire to resist the compulsive act. Indeed, they can control the urge and resist, at least for a short time. Later, the person may just give in and go with it.

In as few as 6 percent of those diagnosed with OCD, compulsions occur without accompanying obsessions. When the two components occur together, as they do in about 70 percent of the cases, it appears that the obsession is causally related to the compulsive act.[34] As a result, the content of the obsession is the source of the urge to perform the act. Two basic forms of compulsions were identified by Akhter and his colleagues as *yielding* and *controlling*.

Yielding Compulsions

Yielding compulsions are the most common type, accounting for 61 percent of Akhter's sample. In these cases, an obsessive thought drives the person to perform some act. For example, one of Akhter's patients, a clerk, had an obsessive thought that he had an important document in one of his pockets. Although he rationally knew this was not true, he felt compelled to, and did, repeatedly check his pocket. The most common type of the yielding compulsions is hand washing. This activity is typically associated with obsessions relating to dirt, germs, or, more generally, fear of contamination and ultimately contracting a disease.

Compulsive hand washing can be exceedingly disruptive, time consuming, and even painful when carried to the proportions often described. Issacs Marks of Maudsley Hospital in London relates a case of a woman who washed her hands up to 100 times a day.[35] She spent hours each day at the sink and her hands became raw and bleeding. Her fear of contamination also required her to use numerous bottles of disinfectant and bars of soap. When the cost of these items exceeded her available income, she resorted to shoplifting them. Finally caught for shoplifting, she was taken to the police station where they tried unsuccessfully to fingerprint her. She had virtually scrubbed off her fingerprints!

An interesting and illustrative sidelight of this case demonstrates the irrationality of compulsive acts and how some can be highly specific. Although this lady washed her hands almost continuously, she would not wash the rest of her body or bathe for weeks at a time. Her body odor was described as unbearable to others around her, but it did not bother her at all.

Controlling Compulsions

The less frequent controlling compulsions (6 percent) take a different form but can be as intense and limiting as those of yielding. These are acts that are performed to allow the individual to control or to resist an obsessive urge without giving in to it. In other cases, the act serves to prevent some other incident from occurring (at least in the person's mind). In many cases, these are like superstitious rituals. An example of a preventive type of controlling compulsion was described by Cammer.[36] This case concerned a lady who felt compelled to touch her venetian blinds four times and then all her pieces of art five times. Her reason for this touching was that it protected her brother from harm. The fact that he always came home safely proved to her that the touching ritual worked. She also admitted that if she did not go through with the ritual, she started to stutter.

Another way of categorizing compulsions is by separating them according to the form of the act itself: what the patient does. Two basic types include the majority of cases: *checkers* and *cleaners*.

The lady just described who compulsively washed her hands was an example of a cleaner. However, not all cleaners are as specific as she nor is the cleaning restricted to washing oneself. Also, as noted previously, cleaning compulsions typically involve obsessive fears of dirt and disease. And, like the phobias, compulsive cleaners may go to great lengths to avoid becoming contaminated. Since contact with other parts of the environment and other people is virtually impossible to avoid, the cleaner will never successfully avoid all "contamination." This then seems to compel them to attempt to restore themselves, or the objects or persons with which they are concerned, to a state of cleanliness, which obviously is an impossible task.[37] In some of the more extreme cases, the attempted avoidance of potential contaminants and the continuous cleaning can be as debilitating as agoraphobia, leaving the person housebound. Even worse than having agoraphobia, however, is the realization that the person has no really safe places; dirt and germs are carried in the very air.

Illustrative of this restriction is the following situation that was described by Rachman and Hodgson:[38]

> A 38-year-old mother of one child had been obsessed by a fear of contamination for over 20 years. Her concern with the possibility of being infected by germs resulted in washing and cleaning rituals that invaded all aspects of her life.

Her child was restrained in one room which was kept entirely germ free. She opened and closed all doors with her feet in order to avoid contaminating her hands. (p. 111)

Compulsive checking involves stereotyped acts carried out with the expressed purpose, on the part of the checker, of ensuring the safety, security, or well-being of oneself, others, or possessions, or to verify the accuracy or security of situations or information.[39] Such checking rituals are seen as preventive of some future or potential problem or disaster.

The clerk who checked for the nonexistent document and the lady who counted her venetian blinds were examples of compulsive checkers. Other common checking compulsions involve persons who check with the police or the newspaper after driving to ensure that they had not caused an accident. Others check repeatedly all windows, water and gas taps, light switches, electric plugs, and doors, for hours before retiring each night. For many checkers and cleaners, though not all, the carrying out of the rituals tends to reduce a felt discomfort and/or anxiety. However, the emotional reduction is not long lasting and the discomfort will recur later.

Compulsive Slowness

Another variant of compulsive behavior is compulsive slowness, or as it has been termed by Rachman and Hodgson, *primary obsessive slowness*.[40] This rare condition is characterized by the individual's taking virtually hours to complete relatively simple tasks, such as getting dressed, washing, putting things away, and the like. Because it takes the better part of a whole day to prepare to leave home, these persons are largely nonfunctional.

Marks described a typical patient of his who would begin preparation for his doctor's appointment the day before it was scheduled.[41] He needed this time because it took five hours to get ready. Similarly, another patient described by Rachman and Hodgson would have to start his preparation to leave at 3 or 4 o'clock in the morning in order to arrive at work by 10 o'clock.

Since preparation of a meal took so long, he ate at a restaurant. About 9 o'clock in the evening, he would begin preparation for bed which he would finally complete around midnight.

These agonizingly slow processes obviously take the vast majority of the waking hours, leaving no time for other pursuits such as employment. Such compulsively slow behavior appears similar to the other compulsions but is also different in several ways. Although the person persists at tasks, the persistence is not typically accompanied by obsessive thoughts. Nor when prompted or pushed to hurry is there the felt anxiety or discomfort experienced by checkers and cleaners when their routines are interrupted.

Also unlike other compulsive individuals, these slow obsessionals are hard pressed to give reasons for their slowness, such as fears or obsessive urges. Rather, it appears to be more of a generalized meticulousness and concern with getting things just right.[42] Although the majority of their lives are taken up with this slow, meticulous behavior, they can talk, walk, and eat at a normal pace. Owing to these differences from other compulsives, there is some question whether they should be classified as obsessive-compulsive at all.[43]

Prevalence and Onset of OCD

Obsessions and compulsions of the proportions described here are apparently relatively rare. Paul Emmelkamp suggested that the general population prevalence is only .05 percent.[44] However, the more recent national survey puts the prevalence at any one time at 1.3 percent to 2 percent. However it is estimated that over the full life span, between 2 and 3 percent of the adult population may experience OCD.[45] This makes them similar in prevalence to panic disorder.

Onset of the obsessive-compulsive disorders can occur at almost any age, with some being documented as early as four years of age, but most starting in late adolescence and early adulthood. The typical onset is in the early 20s and, by age 30, nearly three fourths have developed their symptoms.

In contrast to most other anxiety disorders, males are as likely as females to develop OCD. However, the type of disorder developed may be gender-related. Rachman and his colleagues found that although males and females are equally distributed among compulsive checkers, females clearly predominated among cleaners. This relationship, according to Rachman, supports his view that cleaning compulsions are very similar to phobias where females also are overrepresented.

To explain this gender difference, Emmelkamp goes beyond Rachman's explanation to explain the preponderance of female cleaners.[46] He believes that since females are typically responsible for maintaining the household and therefore cleaning, they would be more likely to develop cleaning compulsions, an overreaction to their domain of responsibility. On the other hand, behaviors associated with checking should have no particular gender-role relatedness and, accordingly, there is no gender difference in prevalence of checkers. Because of the relative rarity of the obsessive-compulsive disorders, sufficient study has not yet been done to clearly delineate the full reasons behind these differences.

Theories of Obsessive-Compulsive Disorder

Among the anxiety disorders, OCD can be the most severe, crippling, and the most resistant to treatment. Although the anxiety experienced does not appear to be any more intense than that seen in other disorders, for many, the obsessive and ritualistic behavior appears to be more resistant to change than are other anxiety-related conditions. Like some other anxiety-related disorders, a large percentage of OCD patients are depressed.[47] As will be discussed in Chapter 10, certain drugs originally designed to treat depression are effective in some OCD cases. The connection between depression and OCD does not seem to mean that they are causally related to one another since, in some cases, depression begins before OCD and for others it is after OCD. As with the other disorders, there are theoretical accounts and supportive data that focus primarily on the psychological processes of the condition while other theory focuses on the biological processes. A variant of each of these approaches will be presented next.

Psychologically Based Theory of OCD

The importance of psychological accounts of OCD stems in part from the fact that there are very few cases of identical twins both of whom have OCD. Thus, there is no evidence of a direct inheritance of OCD. However, as was noted for the other anxiety disorders described, most investigators acknowledge that there may be an inherited tendency toward increased general anxiety and oversensitivity. With this increased potential to be reactive and oversensitive with anxiety, the opportunity is ripe for psychological processes to work to form OCD symptoms.

Another observation that adds credence to this formulation is that many individuals, particularly when under stress, experience obsessive thoughts not unlike those reported by OCD patients. Thus, the strange and even frightening thoughts are not unique to the OCD patient. As part of a long series of investigations, Rachman and de Silva found that normal individuals experienced essentially the same type of obsessional thoughts that the OCD patients did.[48] Further, the thoughts were so similar in content that independent judges were unable to tell whether the thoughts came from patients or from nonpatients. Thus, many people may be capable of experiencing these obsessions. The differences lie in the frequency, duration, and intensity of the thoughts. Patients found the thoughts more distressing and resisted them more than nonpatients. Thus, the thoughts appeared to be more out of their control. Further, it was found that stress tends to increase these obsessional thoughts and stereotypic behaviors in both OCD patients and nonpatients.

For those persons who are particularly upset by these obsessions and who feel that the thoughts are beyond their control, anything that provides some sense of control over the thoughts would be repeated as a control mechanism. It is hypothesized that the repetition of acts that either neutralize the distressing thoughts or eliminate them temporarily would occur with high regularity. This is just what is seen with the compulsive behaviors. At least initially, the behavioral act seems to relieve the person's anxiety or distress over the thought, either by somehow countering the thought or by distracting the person from it temporarily. Since it "works" for them in the short run, they are apt to repeat it each time the thought occurs. This is similar to the process by which the agoraphobic goes to great lengths to ensure that he or she will avoid having a panic attack. Since staying at home reduces the distress and worry over having an attack, staying at home is what the person does repeatedly. Because it works so well, it becomes a very strong "habit" and is exceedingly difficult to break.

In summary, obsessivelike thoughts occur in many people, but especially in those who are anxious and stressed. Some people may be biologically predisposed to be anxious and highly responsive to stresses. If they are particularly upset by these obsessive thoughts and if they find that certain repetitive acts or routines either eliminate or neutralize the distress or anxiety, then these behaviors will be enacted repeatedly whenever the thoughts intrude into their minds. Because they tend to reduce the anxiety, the behaviors are strengthened and themselves become part of the uncontrolled cycle in a way similar to a bad habit that is very difficult to break and that causes the person great distress.

Biologically Based Theory of OCD

One of the most recent biologically based theories of OCD is proposed by Judith Rapoport, Chief of Child Psychiatry at the National Institute of Mental Health.[49] Rapoport's theory begins by noting that two of the main symptoms of OCD involve repetitive cleaning and checking rituals. She was struck by the seeming similarity between the stereotyped behavioral patterns of the OCD patient and the grooming and territorial behaviors seen in many lower animals. These animal behavior patterns are part of their instinctual heritage that has contributed to their specie's survival. The behaviors are now referred to as *fixed action patterns* to imply that they are rigidly programmed action patterns that involve neither learning nor thinking processes. They are said to be *hardwired* or preprogrammed into the animals' brains so that when triggered, they occur as automatic, robotlike rituals. If these patterns were seen outside the appropriate context, they would look very peculiar indeed. For example, stereotyped nest building, courting behaviors, and protective or aggressive behaviors are examples of fixed action patterns.

Rapoport further supports her biological theory of OCD with the observation that this disorder often occurs in association with several neurological disorders that develop from lesions (damages) in a part of the brain called the *basal ganglia*. This area in the interior of the brain is, in part, a pathway or "way station" between sensory information coming into the brain and the thinking and behavioral response to that information. Rapoport proposes that perhaps some disturbance or damage to these areas has occurred that releases the stored preprogrammed behavioral routines akin to the fixed action patterns of lower animals. In other words, they have been short-circuited. After the damage to the basal ganglia, it takes relatively little stimulation to elicit the previously inactive fixed action patterns.

As further support for this biological theory, it is noted that the drugs found to be most effective in treating OCD also act on the neurotransmitter substance *serotonin*, the same substance that is most prevalent in the basal ganglia. While some available data can be interpreted as support for this biological theory, it should be noted that all people with movement disorders involving basal ganglia problems do not necessarily have OCD symptoms. Furthermore, all OCD patients do not necessarily have damage to their basal ganglia; only about 58 percent of OCD patients respond positively to the drugs that affect their serotonin systems. As with the other theories, only further scientific investigation can elucidate the true nature of these puzzling behavior and emotional patterns. And, as with the other conditions described, the "truth" of what causes OCD will most likely include some form of biological predisposition to the condition along with certain psychological, stress, or learning experiences.

REFERENCES

1. Robert Burton, *The Anatomy of Melancholy*, 11th ed. (London: Chatto and Windus 1907).
2. Ibid., 28.
3. Ibid., 221–222.
4. Jerome Myers, Myrna Weissman, Gary Tischler, Charles Holzer, III, Philip Leaf, Helen Orvaschel, James Anthony, Jeffrey Boyd, Jack Burke, Morton Kramer, and Roger Stoltzman, "Six Month Prevalence of Psychiatric Disorders in Three Communities," *Archives of General Psychiatry* 41 (1984): 959–967.
5. Centers for Disease Control Vietnam Experience Survey (VES), "Psychosocial Characteristics," *Journal of The American Medical Association* 259 (1988): 2701–2707.
6. Dean Kilpatrick, Benjamin Saunders, Angelynne Amick-McMullan, Connie Best, Lois Veronen, and Heidi Resnick, "Victim and Crime Factors Associated with the Development of Crime-Related Post-Traumatic Stress Disorder," *Behavior Therapy* 20 (1989): 199–214.
7. Stanley Rachman, *Fear and Courage*, 2nd ed. (New York: W. H. Freeman, 1990).
8. John March, "The Nosology of Posttraumatic Stress Disorder," *Journal of Anxiety Disorders* 4 (1990): 61–82.
9. Kilpatrick *et al.*, "Victim and Crime Factors," 199–214.
10. Edna Foa and Michael Kozak, "Emotional Processing of Fear: Exposure to Corrective Information, *Psychological Bulletin* 99 (1986): 20–35.
11. David Barlow, *Anxiety and Its Disorders* (New York: Guilford Press, 1988).
12. William Sanderson and David Barlow, "A Description of DSM-III-Revised Category O Panic Disorder: Characteristics of 100 Patients with Different Levels of Avoidance." Paper presented at the Annual Meetings of the Association for the Advancement of Behavior Therapy, Chicago (November, 1986).
13. American Psychiatric Association, *Diagnostic and Statistical Manual of Mental Disorders*, 3rd ed., rev. (Washington D. C.: Author, 1987).
14. Barlow, *Anxiety and its Disorders*.
15. Dorothy Jean Anderson, Russell Noyes, and Raymond Crowe, "A Comparison of Panic Disorder and Generalized Anxiety Disorder," *American Journal of Psychiatry* 141 (1984): 572–575.
16. E. H. Uhlenhuth, M. B. Balter, G. D. Mellinger, I. Cisin, and J. Clinthorne,

"Symptom Checklist Syndromes in the General Population: Correlations with Psychotherapeutic Drug Use," *Archives of General Psychiatry* 40 (1983): 1167–1173.

17. Barlow, *Anxiety and Its Disorders*.
18. Dorothy Jean Anderson, Russell Noyes, and Raymond Crowe, "A Comparison of Panic Disorder and Generalized Anxiety Disorder," *American Journal of Psychiatry* 141 (1984): 572–575.
19. Dan Blazer, Dana Hughes, and Linda George, "Stressful Life Events and the Onset of a Generalized Anxiety Syndrome," *American Journal of Psychiatry* 144 (1987): 1178–1183.
20. Raymond Crowe, Russell Noyes, David Pauls, and Don Slymen, "A Family Study of Panic Disorder," *Archives of General Psychiatry* 40 (1983).
21. Svenn Torgersen, "Genetic Factors in Anxiety Disorders," *Archives of General Psychiatry* 40 (1983): 1085–1089.
22. American Psychiatric Association, *Diagnostic and Statistical Manual*.
23. S. Akhter, N. N. Wig, V. K. Varma, D. Pershad, and S. K. Verma, "A Phenomenological Analysis of Symptoms in Obsessive-Compulsive Neurosis," *British Journal of Psychiatry* 127 (1975): 342–348.
24. Ibid.
25. Paul Emmelkamp and H. Wessels, "Flooding in Imagination vs. Flooding *in Vivo:* A Comparison With Agoraphobics," *Behaviour Research and Therapy* 13 (1975): 7–16.
26. Amos Welner, Theodore Reich, Eli Robins, Roberta Fishman, and Thomas Van Doren, "Obsessive-Compulsive Neurosis: Record, Follow-up and Family Studies. I. Inpatient Record Study," *Comprehensive Psychiatry* 17 (1976): 527–539.
27. Akhter *et al.*, "A Phenomenological Analysis," 342–348.
28. Stanley Rachman and Ray Hodgson, *Obsessions and Compulsions* (Englewood Cliffs, N.J.: Prentice-Hall, 1980).
29. S. Akhter *et al.*, 342–348.
30. Ibid.
31. Ibid.
32. Ibid.
33. Rachman and Hodgson, *Obsessions and Compulsions*.
34. Welner *et al.*, "Obsessive-compulsive neurosis," 527–539.
35. Isaac Marks, *Living with Fear* (New York: McGraw-Hill, 1978).
36. L. Cammer, *Freedom from Compulsion* (New York: Simon & Schuster, 1976).
37. Rachman and Hodgson, *Obsessions and Compulsions*.
38. Ibid., 111.
39. Ibid.
40. Ibid.
41. Marks, *Living with Fear*.
42. Rachman and Hodgson, *Obsessions and Compulsions*.
43. Ibid.

44. Emmelkamp and Wessels, "Flooding in Imagination," 7–16.
45. Lee Robins, J. E. Helzer, Myrna Weissman, Helen Orvaschel, E. Gruenberg, Jack Burke, and D. A. Regier, "Lifetime Prevalence of Specific Psychiatric Disorders in Three Sites," *Archives of General Psychiatry* 41 (1984): 949–958.
46. Emmelkamp and Wessels, "Flooding in Imagination," 7–16.
47. Barlow, *Anxiety and Its Disorders.*
48. Stanley Rachman and P. de Silva, "Abnormal and Normal Obsessions," *Behaviour Research and Therapy* 16 (1978): 233–248.
49. Judith Rapoport, "The Biology of Obsessions and Compulsions," *Scientific American* (March, 1989): 83–89.

Childhood and Adolescent Anxiety Disorders

Like adults, children experience anxiety intensely and frequently enough to qualify for all the anxiety-disorder diagnoses. In many cases, the form of the anxiety disorder is identical or highly similar to that seen in adults. However, there are some differences that need to be taken into account. For example, children's avoidance behaviors may be somewhat different from that of adults because of their lesser mobility. Parents often force children to go places where they do not want to go; they have fewer choices.

Also, when examining children's fear and anxiety, the professional must be careful not to ascribe normal, age-related anxiety to an anxiety disorder. Most all children become fearful and avoidant of strangers in the first year of life and they become particularly fearful of leaving their parents or close family members at about one year. As noted in Chapter 2, a number of fears seem to emerge at various ages and then, for the most part, decline as the child continues to develop. Unless these fears become all consuming to the child or do not diminish with age

as expected, they should not be considered fear or anxiety disorders. On the other hand, if the anxiety reactions do persist well
beyond that expected for their age, they can then be classified
according to the anxiety-disorder categories specific to children
or they may be classified into the anxiety disorders previously
described for adults in Chapters 4, 5, and 6. Examples of such
disorders in children will be described in the second part of this
chapter.

Among the ways in which children and adolescents with
anxiety disorders are similar to adults with similar disorders is
that both tend to experience depression. A study by Strauss and
colleagues at the University of Pittsburgh School of Medicine
found that 28 percent of a group of children and adolescents
who were anxiety disordered also were clinically depressed.[1] In
a subsequent study, Strauss found that the depression was
much more likely in the children who were older than 12 years
than in those who were younger than 12 years.[2]

Although children and adolescents can experience the same
disorders as adults, they also display some other patterns somewhat specific to them because of their unique developmental
and life situations. However, as we will see, they clearly have
variants similar or identical to those found with adults. The
specific childhood and adolescent categories include: *overanxious
disorder, avoidant disorder,* and *separation anxiety disorder.* Also included with these categories is a description of *school phobia* or
school refusal as it is sometimes called.

SPECIFIC CHILDHOOD ANXIETY DISORDERS

Overanxious Disorder

The overanxious child or adolescent is characterized by
chronic and excessive worry and fearful behavior. Although
similar in many ways to phobias, the anxiety or fear expressed is
not focused on any specific object or situation nor is it a specific
reaction to some life changes or events. Typically, the child will

worry about future events, exams, being injured, being included with other children, chores to be done, and if he or she will do well enough on whatever task. In these children, there is often an element of perfectionistic tendencies, obsessional self-doubts, conformity, and approval-seeking from others, along with concern over what others think of them. This chronic worry results in continuous states of ANS activation, including feelings of a lump in the throat, headache, stomachache, nausea, "nerves," and difficulty falling asleep. Behaviorally, the child may exhibit such nervous habits as nail biting, restlessness, and hair pulling.

This overanxious condition then has features similar to generalized anxiety disorder, and simple and social phobia. The overanxious child is ripe to develop numerous specific and social fears that work into the more general pattern of excessive concern with possible dangers. But if this overanxiousness persists into adulthood, it may become either GAD or social phobia.[3] Available figures concerning the overall prevalence of this disorder among preadolescent children show it to affect about 2.9 percent of young children and, contrary to other anxiety disorders, males were found to predominate nearly 2 to 1 over females. Data from broad normative samples including adolescents do not exist, so it is unknown just when or how this chronic worrying begins. However, it is known that such children are typically not brought to clinics for treatment until they are about 13 years old.[4] Perhaps by this age, it is clear to parents that the worry is beyond what might be expected for children and that it is not likely to go away on its own. Thus, treatment may be seen as necessary to further the child's social development.

Cindy is a typical overanxious child. At age 11, Cindy was described by her parents as a "good girl," always helpful, overconscientious, and concerned with "doing it right." However, she also seemed to lack confidence in that she repeatedly sought help and reassurance. She was also characterized as sickly, having frequent trips to the doctor's office, including one to the emergency room when she experienced dizziness, faintness, and shortness of breath. She thought she was having a heart attack. Cindy was always highly concerned with safety issues and would occasionally panic over them. For example, one day she panicked over the "possibility" that a tornado might hit and insisted that the family enter the storm shelter.[5]

Avoidant Disorder

Avoidant disorder in children and adolescents involves persistent withdrawal from contact with strangers to the extent that it impairs or prevents relationships with peers. When confronting a stranger, the child becomes essentially mute or inarticulate. Such children typically lack self-confidence and social assertiveness and may express a great desire for attention and affection from family members.

Fear of strangers is, of course, a normal part of development that most young children go through. However, in most cases, this normal fear begins during the first year of life, having an average onset of about eight months of age.[6] Typically, it begins to diminish by the end of the first year and, for most, is gone by the second year of age. A diagnosis of avoidant disorder is only considered after the intense fear of strangers has persisted well past the normal developmental phase, roughly up to two and one-half years of age. Also, it must be shown that the avoidance is interfering with the child's social development and peer relations and, by the teen years, affects interactions with the opposite sex. Prevalence data suggest that this disorder is more common in girls than in boys. Further, it is often found in association with other childhood anxiety disorders, such as overanxious disorder. However, the prevalence of overanxious disorder is particularly unclear since a recent study by Anderson and colleagues was unable to find any children so classified in their broad-scale epidemiologic study of preadolescent children.[7]

In cases in which the condition does exist and if it were to persist into adulthood, it may be considered in another category of avoidant personality disorder, or social phobia, whichever appears to apply. The following case of Avery, described by Robert G. Meyer of the University of Louisville, illustrates the features of social avoidance:[8]

> [When Avery was] three years of age, . . . [his] mother could see that his social development was lagging behind [that of] the other children. He would become upset . . . and cling to her anytime they were outside the house. When anyone outside the family would try to converse with him or encourage him to play with others, he also became upset. Their pediatrician encouraged Avery's mother to enroll him in a day care program to encourage him [to play] with other children. Avery accepted this with reluctance but still maintained much of his avoidant, solitary activity while at day care. He would consent to go, at most, three days a week.
>
> Part of Avery's reticence was due to his shyness about having been born with a short leg and [his fear of] being teased about it. Having been teased about this in the past made him ever more sensitive to his physical defect.

Separation Anxiety Disorder and School Phobia

Separation anxiety, like the two previous categories of childhood and adolescent anxiety disorder, is at some point a normal expectation in children's developmental experiences. Anxiety at being separated from family becomes classified as a disorder only when it is severe and persists beyond what is expected for a child's normal age and expected developmental level. Separation anxiety disorder is characterized by excessive anxiety to the point of panic when a child is separated from parents or parent figures, from home, or from familiar surroundings.[9] The child will typically refuse to visit or stay overnight with friends, run errands, attend camps or school. This latter situation pertaining to school has been referred to as *school refusal* or *school phobia* and will be considered separately.

When anticipating being separated, the child typically clings to the parents and complains of numerous physical symptoms, such as headache, stomachache, and nausea, and may actually vomit. When children with separation anxiety are separated from parents, they become obsessed with worries and fears of accidents that might befall themselves or their parents.

This generalized anxiety, with its cognitive (worry), behavioral (clinging and refusal), and physiological (aches and pains) manifestations, appears to be a form of phobia—a phobia of being left, of illness, or injury occurring either to themselves or to their families. For younger children, the fears are quite general and nonspecific. As children age, their fears become more specific, often centering on concerns of danger and death. Furthermore, these children often have a variety of other fears, such as animals, monsters in the night, being kidnapped, and dying. In sum, it is a rather generalized phobic reaction to many situations, particularly involving being separated. As such, it is akin to adult manifestations of agoraphobia. Consequently, this generalized fear, along with avoidance of being out alone, may result in somewhat of a diagnostic dilemma concerning whether to call it a phobic disorder or separation anxiety disorder. This issue becomes particularly pertinent with school refusal or school phobia.

As one might expect, sleep disturbance is not uncommon, often involving insomnia and nightmares. These experiences may well explain why the child often attempts to sleep with his or her parents. When separated, older children may become extremely homesick, may yearn to return home, and may become preoccupied with fantasies of returning. But older children may deny needing the parent on account of their embarrassment, even though their behavior belies their lack of concern.

Although broad prevalence figures for adolescents are not available, separation anxiety disorder was found in one study to include as many as 3.5 percent of preadolescent children. The one study available also found girls to predominate 2 to 1 over boys.[10]

Fear of the dark and possible scary imaginary creatures that might be there are common themes of these children's fears. Depression, along with chronic complaining, statements that no one loves them, and the wish that they were dead are often seen as well.

When the child becomes fearful of separation, refusal to go to school often follows. School refusal may represent a case of school phobia. However, often the school refusal is part of the larger picture of separation anxiety; that is, it is not school that they fear but separation from parents. In keeping with recommendations of DSM-III-R, it would seem more appropriate to retain the term *school phobia* for those cases in which the anxiety and fear reactions occur on account of school *per se*. When school refusal is due to fear of being separated more generally, *separation anxiety* is the more appropriate term. School refusal children will attempt to avoid school by convincing their parents that they are ill and should be allowed to stay home. Complaints typically include stomachache, headache, not feeling well, and the like. The anticipatory anxiety generated by the thought of having to go to school may, in fact, cause the child to have a stomachache or to vomit, which, of course, is rather convincing to the parents.

Physical complaints are typically most pronounced in the morning, before school. If allowed to stay home, the child will feel better by early afternoon, after the threat of having to go to school has passed.[11] However, the "illness" will return the next morning or the next school day. Also, such complaints are more likely to occur on Mondays and diminish by the weekend.

As with other phobias, school phobia does not go away with reassurance or with minor changes in the school environment. Although school phobia can begin at virtually any grade level including college, it appears to peak during periods of major traumas and transitions, such as when first beginning school (5–8 years of age) and junior high or high school (11–14 years of age).[12]

Although prevalence rates are difficult to interpret because of the possible confusion with separation anxiety, school phobia has been estimated to involve between 1 and 2 percent of school-aged children.[13] The following case described by Price and Lynn, illustrates the fact that the distinction between separation anxiety disorder, school phobia, and even simple phobia is often difficult or impossible to make. In fact, in many cases, these conditions may not be separable at all.[14]

> Jeannie, a normal 7 year old, had attended school only 5 days out of the past two months. She "felt bad," had stomach aches, headaches, vomiting, and diarrhea. However, she was considerably better on weekends. Just prior to the onset of her anxiety, she had been hospitalized for a severe infection where her mother let it be known that she feared that Jeannie might die. Later, Jeannie's grandmother did die during surgery. Jeannie then learned that she had to return to the hospital for a tonsillectomy. With these prior hospital episodes so prominent in her mind, she was openly fearful of dying and, by then, would not leave home without her parents. To make matters worse, at school, her teacher became ill, the substitute teacher yelled at Jeannie and embarrassed her to the point that at lunch she called home to have her mother come get her.

By the time of the episode in which the teacher yelled at her, Jeannie had developed a fear of dying and of hospitals (simple phobia), she was fearful of being left by her parents (separation anxiety disorder), and she began to avoid school on account of numerous physical complaints (school phobia). Jeannie's behavior could have qualified her for any or all of these diagnoses.

Prevalence of Specific Childhood Anxiety Disorders

The exact prevalence of these child and adolescent anxiety disorders is not known. However, in a recent study, Javad Kashani and Helen Orvaschel of the University of Missouri examined a randomly selected group of 210 children, aged 8 through 17 years and administered to them an anxiety-disorders interview. They found that 21 percent of their sample had one or more anxiety disorders.[15] Of those with an anxiety disorder, 36 percent had more than one diagnosis, with the most frequent diagnoses being separation anxiety and overanxious disorders.

The type of symptoms experienced was found to be related to the age of the children. As we noted in Chapter 2 in the discussion of general fears, younger children were troubled mostly by bad dreams, separation from family, presence of strangers, and were more often sick to their stomachs. Older children in their teens were more concerned with social fears, past imperfections, and tended to worry a great deal.

The finding by Kashani and Orvaschel that 21 percent of children and adolescents had anxiety disorders was similar to figures found among adults, where anxiety disorders were found to be the most frequent of all mental disorders.[16] Also, like adult samples, girls were more frequently diagnosed as having anxiety disorders than were boys at all age levels. Thus, to the extent that this study is representative of children throughout the United States, childhood anxiety is at least as frequent as that found in adults.

ANXIETY DISORDERS IN CHILDREN

Simple Phobia in Children

Like adults, many children experience specific or simple phobias. It is estimated that in the neighborhood of 2 percent of children have clinical-level phobias.[17,18] The most common childhood phobias are of animals (dogs, cats, mice, spiders, and the like) and of illness or injury. Even though these fears and phobias are relatively common among young children, most outgrow them or perhaps overcome them through experience or finding out that the objects or animals are not as harmful as they feared they would be. However, virtually all adults with animal phobias, for example, acquired them during childhood, usually around age 4. Thus, if these phobic fears are not treated or do not go away early on, they are unlikely to simply disappear on their own.

Jerry, an active 10-year-old, had recently moved outside of town with his mother and sister. From his new home, he had to walk up a long driveway to get to the main road to catch the school bus. At first, this was no problem, he enjoyed playing along the way. However, Jerry soon became aware that a number of large dogs roamed the neighborhood. After these dogs chased Jerry one day, he became frightened and, from then on, was unwilling to walk to or from the bus stop alone. Further, he felt he was no longer able to play outside alone or even walk around outside his house. In order to get Jerry to the bus, his mother had to drive him to the bus stop where he waited in the car until the bus came. She had to be at the bus stop with the car when he came home or he would not get off the bus. While Jerry's fear had become quite limiting, it was also of interest in its specificity. He had his own dog that had been a pet for many years and it did not bother him, except on occasion if it growled at him. His fear was of large, strange dogs only.

In our discussion in Chapter 2 of the ways in which fears and phobias can be acquired, we noted that information or misinformation could lead to such fears. The following cases illustrate the development in a young adolescent of just such a simple phobia: that of contracting AIDS. Recall that the feared disease or *nosophobia* seems to change over time. Today, the concern with AIDS, along with the prevention-oriented publicity that is seen, has brought AIDS into focus as the newest phobic disease target.

Illustrating this nosophobia, Lewin and Williams recently reported two such cases in the *British Journal of Psychiatry*.[19] One case involved a 13-year-old child who became unduly concerned with contracting AIDS to the extent that he was preoccupied with thoughts of contracting the disease and became involved in continual intense hand washing to cleanse himself. He also "avoided television lest AIDS or homosexuality was mentioned or intimate physical contact was portrayed" (p. 823). This phobic and obsessive behavior developed following a school biology class devoted to "germs" and was coincident in time with a large-scale media campaign to inform the public of AIDS.

A second phobic case was similar in that its victim, aged 12, had become fearful each night at bedtime and was unable to sleep alone. He confided to his parents that he was exceedingly fearful of contracting AIDS. His fear evolved from his conviction that it was inevitable that he would catch AIDS. He knew that he was ignorant of AIDS and he took to heart a television publicity piece imploring people: "Don't die of ignorance."[20] Since he knew he was ignorant of it, he felt sure that he would contract it and die.

Childhood Obsessive-Compulsive Disorder

Like the phobias, OCD very often begins in childhood or adolescence and persists into adulthood.[21,22] In fact, one half of all cases develop by the end of the teens. The youngest age at which OCD has been documented thus far is 3 years. One such child at 3 repetitively circled manhole covers on the streets and became very upset when this routine was interrupted. Another at age 3 was noted to have walked only on the edges of tiles and by age 7 had become a light switch and door checker.[23]

An interesting difference found between OCD and the other anxiety disorders concerns the gender distributions. In most other disorders, except as noted for overanxious disorder, females predominate. Among all OCD types for adults there is no gender difference in prevalence.[24] Among children with OCD, boys may be overrepresented.

The gender differences also vary by disorder type. For example, among obsessionals who do not have compulsive rituals, males predominate, while cleaners are largely females. Furthermore, OCD begins considerably earlier in males than in females, particularly for checkers, where the average age of onset for males is 14 years, whereas it is 21 years for females.[25] These differences suggest to some researchers that OCD may be a quite different disorder from the other anxiety disorders.[26] However, noting the case on AIDS phobia cited previously, in some cases there does appear to be a relationship between irrational fears, particularly of cleanliness and contracting illness, and obsessive and compulsive behaviors.

OCD is as debilitating for children as it is for adults. When fully into their rituals, children may be unable to engage in other activities, including school. This is what happened to the 13-year-old girl whose case was described in the American Psychiatric Association's Diagnostic Casebook.[27]

> She described her compulsions as: ". . . really stupid and they didn't make any sense; but I'm still gonna have to do it and, it was sort of like being scared of what would happen if I didn't do it" (p. 309). This part of the problem stemmed from her fear of dirt and germs. When she believed that germs were on her clothes, she would shake them for a half an hour. To clean her hands, she would scrub them with rubbing alcohol until they bled. This would take as much as 6 hours a day to clean.
>
> Her obsessions involved set plans in her mind of how to deal with certain words that set off her cleaning. She devised mental rituals to cancel or neutralize these words such as repeating the phrase "soap and water" or the number 3. These mental rituals, like superstitious behaviors, were performed to prevent bad things from happening to others she cared about if she didn't do them. This overconcern extended to the case that she worried that something she did would cause her 83-year-old grandmother to get sick. Intellectually, she knew that these thoughts were irrational, but emotionally she was scared they were true.

Panic Disorder and Agoraphobia in Children

Young children are not immune to the terrifying effects of panic disorder and panic can lead them to agoraphobia as well as it can with adults. The study mentioned in Chapter 6, conducted by Jennifer Lee Macaulay and myself, found as many as 5 percent of our adolescent sample to experience severe enough panics to appear to qualify for the diagnosis of panic disorder. Of these panickers, the average age at which they recalled experiencing their first panic was 13 years, indicating that one half began before 13 years of age.[28]

Increasingly, more cases are being recorded in psychological and psychiatric reports documenting that even younger children develop PD. Some children as young as 5 years of age experience the full syndrome of panic disorder. Further, many also display agoraphobic avoidance similar to that seen in adults.[29,30] James Ballenger and colleagues at the Medical University of South Carolina recently described the following two cases of Ann and Cathy:

> At 8 years of age, Ann developed abdominal pains along with non-specific fear reactions when in crowded places. She avoided any activity with family or at school that required her to go into crowded places. Particularly when in a crowded place, Ann would experience the typical panic symptoms of heart palpitations, shortness of breath, pains, and feeling she was losing control. These attacks would occur as often as twice a day when she was away from home. She would frequently call from school asking to be taken home. Due to her stomach pains and avoidance of crowds, she refused to eat at the school cafeteria resulting in the loss of 5 pounds within three months.

> Cathy had always had problems with separation from her parents and avoided spending the night with friends. At age 11, following a move to a new school, she began to develop stomach pains. At school she experienced panic attacks consisting of feelings that she was going to die, dizziness, sweating, trembling, and so on. Her agoraphobia presented a difficult situation for her as she did not

want to be left alone, but when she accompanied her mother on errands she would panic in stores. She had no refuge except to be at home with her mother.

These two cases of children with panic disorder illustrate a commonly observed occurrence—that panic attacks often are associated with separation anxiety. In each of these cases, the child could also be diagnosed as having separation anxiety disorder and school phobia. The frequent complaint of stomachaches and pains, as seen in both of these cases, is almost universal among children with school phobia.

Posttraumatic Stress Disorder in Children

Children, like adults, who are exposed to severe stressors and traumatic events develop the full complement of symptoms of PTSD described in Chapter 6. Although PTSD in children has been studied somewhat less than it has in adults, information is accumulating. The major stressors for children include natural disasters (floods and tornados), physical and sexual abuse, and experiencing and witnessing violence. Although figures are not available for comparison, it would seem reasonable to assume that children exposed to severe stressors might be even more affected than adults. Children have fewer experiences to relate stressors to, fewer personal and stress-coping skills, and they are much less likely to have any degree of control over the situation or their own reactions to the situation.

Childhood stress responses are reported to occur as young as 2 years of age. In one tragic case, a 2-year-old child was abducted from his father and stepmother by his biological mother. The abducting mother returned the child within five weeks, however, because of his extreme emotional symptoms that included sleep difficulties (nightmares, frequent awakenings, night terrors, and screaming), eating difficulties, and loss of toilet habits. These symptoms persisted for a year after his return and were only resolved with treatment.[31]

A recent study took advantage of a major tragedy to gain

information on childhood PTSD. In February, 1984, a sniper opened fire on a playground full of children in a Los Angeles elementary school. The children were pinned down for several hours, some hiding behind trees or trash cans, others simply lying still on the ground. Thirteen children were physically injured and one was killed.[32] One month following this assault, a team of clinical researchers interviewed and diagnosed 159 children, some of whom were on the playground, others who were in the school, and yet others who were out of school at the time. Their examination of the children showed that the closer the children were to actual tragedy, the more severe their PTSD symptoms. This, as would be expected, is the same result as was found for war veterans. The greater the degree of combat experience, the greater the PTSD. For women who were physically assaulted, those who believed their lives were in mortal danger were the more severely affected.

The group of symptoms that most clearly identified children affected with PTSD were intrusive thoughts and images regarding reexperiencing the event, the wish to avoid feelings, and loss of interest in previously enjoyable activities. Also characteristic of the more severely affected children was experiencing bad dreams, having difficulty attending school, and feeling guilty for having survived. Note that these symptoms are virtually identical to those experienced by combat soldiers.

One child's distress from this incident is described below:

> Leah at age seven had been on the playground that day. Three months following the incident, her teacher had become concerned that this previously well-behaved good student had changed. She began to bicker with others, withdrew from her friends, and lost interest in her schoolwork. She startled when the PA system came on or when someone shouted in the classroom. Following the incident, she had displayed similar behavior at home. Leah had become clinging, fearful, and moody, and she regularly asked to sleep with her parents. She experienced nightmares about her or her family being shot, was chronically

tired, had multiple physical complaints, and showed little interest in her usual games. Now she played nurse games in which a nurse bandaged an injured person. Leah recalled vividly images of an injured girl lying on the ground bleeding. These images interfered with her attention at other times such as in class when she would lose track of what was being said. She avoided the playground and areas close to where the shooting took place and was particularly frightened on Fridays, the day of the week when the shooting happened.

Leah was clearly experiencing most all of the symptoms characteristic of adult PTSD. One difference between children and adults is that the experience of flashbacks does not seem to occur with children. Also characteristic of children, Leah incorporated elements of the trauma into her play.

SUMMARY AND CONCLUSIONS

The descriptions of anxiety disorders in children presented in this chapter indicate that age does not protect one from the disabling effects of anxiety disorders. Although the form may vary somewhat, each of the anxiety disorders are experienced by children. In addition, there are anxiety disorders specific to children that are related in some cases to what might be considered lags in social development. The overanxious, avoidant, and separation anxiety disorders all consist of behaviors and emotional expressions that are quite normal and expected at some point in a child's development. Although these fear-related behaviors can be intense and distressing to parents, they should not be considered psychological disorders until it is shown that they are not only persistent but that they persist well beyond the expected time for the specific developmental state. It should be remembered that the range of normal development is quite broad.

REFERENCES

1. Cyd Strauss, Cynthia Last, Michel Hersen, and Alan Kazdin, "Association between Anxiety and Depression in Children and Adolescents with Anxiety Disorders," *Journal of Abnormal Child Psychology* 16 (1988): 57–68.
2. Cyd Strauss, Cynthia Lease, Cynthia Last, and Greta Francis, "Overanxious Disorder: An Examination of Developmental Differences," *Journal of Abnormal Child Psychology* 16 (1988): 433–443.
3. American Psychiatric Association, *Diagnostic and Statistical Manual of Mental Disorders*, 3rd ed., rev. (Washington D. C.: Author, 1987).
4. Ibid.
5. Robert Carson, James Butcher, and James Colman, *Abnormal Psychology and Modern Life*, 8th ed. (Boston: Scott Foresman, 1989).
6. B. R. McCandless and R. Trotter, *Children: Behavior and Development*, 3rd ed. (New York: Holt, Rinehart and Winston, 1977).
7. Jessie C. Anderson, Sheila Williams, Rob McGee, and Phil Silva "DSM-III Disorders in Preadolescent Children," *Archives of General Psychiatry*, 44, (1987), 69–76.
8. Robert G. Meyer, *Cases in Developmental Psychology and Psychopathology* (Needham Heights, Mass.: Allyn and Bacon, 1989).
9. American Psychiatric Association, *Diagnostic and Statistical Manual*.
10. Jessie C. Anderson, Sheila Williams, Rob McGee, and Phil Silva, "DSM-III Disorders in Preadolescent Children," *Archives of General Psychiatry* 44 (1987): 69–76.
11. Charles Wenar, *Psychopathology from Infancy through Adolescence* (New York: Random House, 1982).
12. Ibid.
13. Ibid.
14. Richard Price and Steven Lynn, *Abnormal Psychology*, 2nd ed. (Chicago: Dorsey Press, 1986).
15. Javad Kashani and Helen Orvaschel, "A Community Study of Anxiety in Children and Adolescents," *American Journal of Psychiatry* 147 (1990): 313–318.
16. Jerome Myers, Myrna Weissman, Gary Tischler, Charles Holzer, III, Philip Leaf, Helen Orvaschel, James Anthony, Jeffrey Boyd, Jack Burke, Morton Kramer, and Roger Stoltzman, "Six Month Prevalence of Psychiatric Disorders in Three Communities, *Archives of General Psychiatry* 41 (1984): 959–967.
17. Anderson *et al.*, "DSM-III Disorders," 69–76.
18. Barbara Melamed and Lawrence Segal, "Children's Reactions to Medical Stressors," in *Anxiety and the Anxiety Disorders*, A. Hussain Tuma and Jack D. Maser, ed. (Hillsdale, N.J.: Lawrence Erlbaum Associates, 1985), 369–388.
19. C. Lewin and R. J. W. Williams, "Fear of AIDS: The Impact of Public Anxiety in Young People," *British Journal of Psychiatry* 153 (1988): 823–824.
20. Ibid., 824.

21. Susan Swedo, Judith Rapoport, Henrietta Leonard, Marge Lenane, and Deborah Cheslow, "Obsessive-Compulsive Disorder in Children and Adolescents Clinical Phenomenology of 70 Consecutive Cases," *Archives of General Psychiatry* 46 (1989): 335–341.

22. William Minnichiello, Lee Baer, Michael Jenike, and Amy Hollond, "Age of Onset of Major Subtypes of Obsessive-Compulsive Disorder," *Journal of Anxiety Disorders* 4 (1990): 147–150.

23. Susan Swedo, Judith Rapoport, Henrietta Leonard, Marge Lenane, and Deborah Cheslow, "Obsessive-Compulsive Disorder in Children and Adolescents Clinical Phenomenology of 70 Consecutive Cases, *Archives of General Psychiatry* 46 (1989): 335–341.

24. Minnichiello *et al.*, "Age of Onset," 147–150.

25. Ibid.

26. Swedo *et al.*, "Obsessive-Compulsive Disorder," 335–341.

27. Robert Spitzer, M. Gibbon, A. Skodol, Janet Williams, and M. First, *DSM-III-R Casebook* (Washington, D.C.: American Psychiatric Association Press, 1987), 309–311.

28. Jennifer Lee Macaulay and Ronald Kleinknecht, "Panic and Panic Attacks in Adolescents," *Journal of Anxiety Disorders* 4 (1989): 221–241.

29. Donna Moreau, Myrna Weissman, and Virginia Warner, "Panic Disorder in Children at High Risk for Depression," *American Journal of Psychiatry* 146 (1989): 1059–1060.

30. James Ballenger, Donald Carek, Jane Steele, and Denise Cornish-McTighe, "Three Cases of Panic Disorder with Agoraphobia in Children, *American Journal of Psychiatry* 146 (1989): 922–924.

31. N. Senior, T. Gladstone, and B. Nurcombe, "Child Snatching: A Case Report," *Journal of the American Academy of Child Psychiatry* 21 (1982): 579–583.

32. Robert Pynoos, Calvin Fredrick, Kathi Nader, William Arroyos, Alan Steinberg, Spencer Eth, Francisco Nunez, and Lynn Fairbanks, "Life Threat and Posttraumatic Stress in School-Age Children, *Archives of General Psychiatry* 44 (1987): 1057–1062.

Treatment Procedures for the Anxiety Disorders

Among the anxiety disorders are some of the most treatable of all psychiatric or psychological conditions. The phobias, and particularly the simple specific phobias and panic disorder, can be successfully treated in the majority of cases. Some reports of simple animal phobias show up to 100 percent treatment effectiveness.[1] Other anxiety-based disorders, however, are more refractory. For example, although numerous successful treatments of obsessive-compulsive disorders have been reported, many other cases have not yielded to current treatment methods.[2]

In this chapter, I will describe some of the most effective psychological procedures that are used for treating the anxiety disorders. The procedures to be described are generically referred to as *behavior therapy*. More recently, with the increasing recognition of the important role played by cognitive or thinking processes in the development of these disorders, the treatment procedures have been expanded to include alterations of thinking patterns and thus are now called *cognitive-behavior therapy* (CBT). In Chapter 9, these treatment procedures are further illustrated by my descriptions of their use with several clinical cases of anxiety disorders and, in Chapter 10, I will conclude and provide an overview of drug treatment for the anxiety disorders.

The treatment procedures to be described are all aimed at uncoupling the ties between situations, including thoughts, and the automatic fear or anxiety responses. These procedures accomplish this uncoupling by focusing on changing the three main response components. Although the several procedures have the same goal of reducing the anxiety or fear, they have different emphases. Some focus on attempting to directly reduce the physiological reactivity by training the anxious person in relaxation. Other procedures focus first on eliminating the avoidance component by ensuring the individual is exposed to the anxiety-provoking situation without allowing escape. Other approaches, focusing on the cognitive component, attempt to restructure or change anxiety-provoking thoughts and self-statements. All these procedures are hypothesized to affect the belief structure of persons with respect to their ability to handle the anxiety-provoking situation and to control themselves while in the presence of the feared or anxiety-provoking situations.

Note that most of the procedures described focus on alleviating only the irrational and debilitating aspects of fear or anxiety responses as seen in the phobias or generalized anxiety. It would make little sense to attempt to eliminate all fear responding! And even if it could be done, it would be highly unadaptive for a person not to respond with some fear to realistic dangers.

A general goal of these procedures is to instill in unduly fearful and anxious persons a sense of confidence that they can cope with the feared situation and develop in them a feeling of personal control over their own fear responding. After describing the various treatments, I will return to this issue in a discussion of possible unifying concepts at the end of this chapter.

TREATMENT PROCEDURES

Systematic Desensitization

Systematic desensitization (SD) was the first of the behavior therapy procedures found effective in treating anxiety-based disorders. Developed by Joseph Wolpe in the 1950s, SD has been proven effective in literally hundreds of experimental investigations.[3] Although evidence of its effectiveness has been demonstrated for most all of the anxiety disorders, SD appears to be most fruitfully applied to the phobias. Consequently, in the following discussions of this technique, simple phobias will be used as the prototypic example.

Wolpe theorized that neurotic disorders (i.e., anxiety based) largely consist of maladaptive anxiety responses being tied to environmental events, such as objects or situations, through the process of classical conditioning.[4] The task of treatment then becomes one of breaking the link between the stimulus that has come to elicit the anxiety and the anxiety response itself. This is accomplished by substituting a new or more adaptive response to the stimulus. To describe this process, Wolpe invoked the principle of *reciprocal inhibition* which states: "If a response inhibiting anxiety can be made to occur in the presence of anxiety-evoking stimuli, it will weaken the bond between these stimuli and anxiety."[5]

A number of responses have been shown to serve this purpose of inhibiting the anxiety response. Among those used are eating, sexual stimulation, assertive behavior (for social anxiety), and relaxation.[6] The response found most useful and versatile and hence most commonly used is relaxation.

The basic goal of SD is to enable the fearful or anxious person to relax in the presence of the anxiety-provoking stimulus. This is done in a stepwise fashion to facilitate the reciprocal inhibition process. The treatment begins by first training the person in deep muscle relaxation. Then, while deeply relaxed, the person imagines various scenes associated with the object or situation that elicits the fear reaction. Each of the steps and processes involved will now be described in greater detail.

Relaxation Training

There are many effective ways to attain a state of relaxation and for the purposes of SD it makes little difference which is used. However, the method most frequently used is one which Wolpe patterned after the progressive relaxation training of Edmund Jacobson.[7] The training proceeds by having the person tense specific muscle groups, one at a time. While tensing the forearm, for example, the person is asked to focus on the sensations of tenseness so they become very familiar with the sensations. Then, after 5 to 7 seconds, the arm is relaxed and the contrast between tension and relaxation is attended to. The alternate tensing-relaxing cycle allows the muscles sort of a running start to relaxing. Once one set of muscles has begun relaxing, it is allowed to continue to relax and another set is introduced with the same sequence of tension-relaxation until the entire body is relaxed.[8]

Although this or any other relaxation procedure is an integral part of SD, deep muscle relaxation is highly therapeutic itself. There is ample evidence that such relaxation, even though directed at the muscles, results in overall diminutions in SNS arousal, including lowered blood pressure, pulse rate, skin conductance, respiration, and the like. Also accompanying the physical relaxation is typically a calming of the person's subjective mental state as well. An adequate level of relaxation can usually be achieved after a couple of weeks of training with daily practice.

The Anxiety Hierarchy

The next step in SD is the construction of a list of situations that cause the person to become anxious or fearful. This list is then graded in terms of the degree to which each situation causes anxiety. The list of situations, ranked in order of anxiety arousal, is called the *anxiety hierarchy*. These are situations to be imagined at a later time while the person relaxes. An example of an anxiety hierarchy constructed for a person fearful of dentistry is shown in Table 12.

The procedure for grading the hierarchy can be facilitated by having the person assign to each situation a number from 0 to 100 to represent the amount of anxiety it causes. These numbers are referred to as *subjective units of disturbance* (SUDS).[9] According to Wolpe, there should be no more than about 10 SUDS

TABLE 12
Anxiety Hierarchy for Dental Phobia

Anxiety–provoking situation	SUD (0–100)
1. Opening a magazine and seeing the word "dentist."	20
2. Calling for an appointment.	25
3. Seeing the calendar that shows only one day left before appointment.	32
4. Driving to the dentist's office.	39
5. Entering the waiting room.	45
6. Hearing the drill sounds while in the waiting room.	54
7. Being taken into the dental chair.	60
8. Seeing the dentist walk in.	68
9. Dentist uses explorer (probe) to examine your teeth.	73
10. Feeling vibrations from the drill on your tooth.	80
11. Seeing the local anesthetic syringe.	90
12. Dentist begins injection.	95

between adjacent items on the hierarchy.[10] That is, there should not be a large jump in anxiety-provoking potential from one item to the next.

The Desensitization Procedure

Once the fearful person has attained skill in deep muscle relaxation and the hierarchy or hierarchies (if more than one is needed) are constructed, the actual desensitization can proceed. As noted previously, the task is to enable the person to imagine the anxiety-provoking situations from the hierarchy while maintaining relaxation. The step in the actual desensitization process is accomplished by having the person deeply relax. Then the therapist begins by presenting the least anxiety-provoking scene from the hierarchy for the person to imagine. For example, from the hierarchy in Table 12 it would be: "Imagine opening a magazine and seeing the word 'dentist.'" If the person then experiences any anxiety, he or she is instructed to signal the therapist, usually by raising a finger. At the signal of felt anxiety, the subject is instructed to stop imagining the word "dentist" and attempt to regain the full state of relaxation. Usually, a neutral or very pleasant scene, determined in advance—such as lying on the beach in the warm sun—is used at this point to facilitate relaxing and to give the subject something peaceful to think about. Once relaxation is regained, the anxiety scene is presented again. Each successive presentation typically results in a reduction in anxiety until the subject is able to remain completely relaxed while visualizing the scene. At this point, the second item is presented until the person masters it. This process is repeated for each item until the subject masters the entire hierarchy with no signs of anxiety.

The critical issue here is not simply that the subject is able to *imagine* the scenes without anxiety, but rather that it is the subject's lack of anxiety response from imagining which carries over to real-life confrontations with the actual feared situations. This carry-over does indeed occur.

The exact mechanism by which the desensitization process works is still a matter of some theoretical controversy. Wolpe contends that it is essentially a counter-conditioning process in which relaxing in the imaginal presence of the fear stimuli inhibits the fear or anxiety response. With repeated pairings of relaxation with the previously fear-provoking stimuli, the relaxation response becomes conditioned to those stimuli, that is, counter-conditioning.

Other researchers have proposed that the anxiety-reducing effects of SD are due to an extinction process; that is, the presentation of the conditioned stimulus (the feared situation) without the experiencing of the unconditioned stimulus, or that which is frightening or aversive. For example, if one were shown a red light, followed by an electric shock, soon the light would become a conditioned stimulus and would cause an anticipatory anxiety response. However, if the light were then repeatedly presented without shock, the anxiety response would eventually diminish and disappear or be extinguished. Although the matter of whether the effectiveness of SD is a result of counter-conditioning, extinction, neither, or both is unclear. It is clear that the process is highly effective for treating fear and anxiety problems.

Variations on the Desensitization Procedures

A number of variations of systematic desensitization procedures have been investigated. These studies have extended the uses and efficiency of SD and have also called into question the need for some of the procedures originally described by Wolpe. One of the first variations introduced was to examine the effectiveness of SD applied to *groups* of fearful persons, all with a common fear or phobia. Following Arnold Lazarus's first demonstration of group desensitization,[11] a number of other investigators found the procedure as effective as when applied individually for treating test anxiety,[12] for social anxiety,[13] for snake phobia,[14] and for spider phobia.[15]

A second variation was the use of *automated* desensitization in which the therapist's presence was not needed.[16] After initially being introduced to the procedure by the therapist, the subject was given relaxation instructions from a prerecorded audio tape recorder. The anxiety hierarchy scenes were also presented on tape. The tape was programmed so that the subject could control which scene was presented, terminate the scene if anxiety was felt, and reset it to repeat scenes. Among the advantages of this type of automated procedure are minimal therapist time required once the procedure is set up, and availability for subjects to conduct their own treatment at home.[17] In a highly innovative study, Donner and Guerney found automated group desensitization to be highly effective as well as efficient in diminishing fears.[18]

Another variation on the standard desensitization procedures was introduced by Marvin Goldfried.[19] Goldfried conceptualized the desensitization process as one in which the patient learns to exercise self-control over his or her anxiety response in the presence of anxiety-provoking stimuli. In this variation, subjects are not instructed to stop visualizing scenes once anxiety is experienced. Rather, they are instructed to continue to imagine the scene and attempt to relax away the tension experienced. By this process, the subjects gain practice in actively controlling, managing, and finally overcoming their own fear reactions.

Goldfried's conceptualization of SD also has theoretical implications. He suggested that the critical process is not just a passive counter-conditioning or extinction but rather an active process of learning to control one's own reaction. Consequently, the attention paid to the graded anxiety hierarchy is seen as less important than the general practice in controlling one's anxiety by using relaxation in any anxiety-related situation.

In vivo desensitization is another variation on the traditional systematic desensitization procedure. In *in vivo* desensitization, the subject confronts the feared situation live or directly, rather than in imagined scenes. Depending on the nature of the stimuli, this direct confrontation can occur in the consulting office, or the individual can be taken, with the therapist, directly into the situation, or clients can conduct the exposure by themselves. The same SD procedure can be used: relaxing, viewing, or experiencing the situation directly until anxiety is felt, and then returning to relaxation. This *in vivo* exposure was also recommended by Goldfried as a situation in which self-control of anxiety could be practiced.

Wolpe recommended the *in vivo* approach, particularly for subjects who are unable to clearly imagine their feared situation and for whom visualization does not generate sufficient anxiety to be realistic.[20] *In vivo* desensitization has been shown to be at least as effective as imagined and when used in conjunction with the imaginal procedures, facilitates the desensitization process.[21]

Although many aspects of SD procedures can be varied and some may not even be necessary, however, one element does seem essential: systematic exposure to the feared stimulus or situation. Whether live or imagined, some exposure to the anxiety-provoking stimuli without the individual experiencing aversive or catastrophic consequences appears to be the common denominator of these treatments.[22] This element of nonreinforced exposure to feared stimuli is the basis for another set of anxiety-reduction treatment procedures: the exposure techniques.

The Exposure Treatments

In contrast to SD, the exposure treatments are designed to generate high levels of anxiety or fear response in the presence of eliciting stimuli. Whether conducted in imagination or *in vivo*, the individual is exposed to his or her anxiety-provoking situation without escaping. The patient experiences the anxiety until it abates, which it invariably does.

The theory supporting the effects of the exposure techniques is that repeated, prolonged exposure to eliciting stimuli results in extinction of the conditioned fear or anxiety response. The process of extinction of fear responses was described in the previous section as an alternate explanation for the effect of SD. Repeated exposure to the eliciting stimulus (CS) without experiencing anticipated negative consequences leads to a reduction and eventual elimination of the automatic or conditioned fear response. After a number of exposures to the previous fear stimulus, the person "learns" that the stimulus no longer has the threat value it once did. For example, an individual may have become phobic of dogs after having been attacked and bitten by one as a child. To treat this phobia with exposure, the person would be exposed to dogs, which initially would elicit considerable anxiety. However, repeated exposure to the dogs, without being bitten again, would result in the extinction of the conditioned anxiety response. The person's repeated exposure would show that the stimulus "dog" is no longer a potential threat or danger.

In addition to the extinction of the CR, another process contributes to the effectiveness of the exposure techniques. Recall from earlier chapters that avoidance of the feared situation prevents extinction from occurring and maintains the fear. Escape or avoidance behavior was said to be reinforced because it removes a person from an unpleasant situation. The exposure techniques also eliminate this component, extinguishing both the conditioned response and the avoidance behavior.

Variations of the Exposure Treatments

There are several variations of how these exposure techniques can be applied. However, all are structured to elicit anxiety or fear in such a way as to facilitate extinction.

Flooding

Flooding involves exposing the subject to the intense anxiety-provoking stimuli. The exposure can be accomplished either through imaginal scenes or by direct, live contact with the anxiety eliciting stimuli. In both cases, the individual is prevented from escaping.

In recent years, flooding has been subjected to an increasing amount of research and application. It and its variants have been found to be highly effective in treating a wide variety of anxiety disorders, including simple phobias, panic disorder, agoraphobia, generalized anxiety disorder, and obsessive-compulsive disorders.[23,24] Indeed, flooding and other forms of exposure have emerged as the treatments of choice in some of the more complex anxiety disorders such as agoraphobia and obsessive-compulsive disorders.

Several procedural variations were found to contribute to the overall effectiveness of the exposure techniques. First, it has been generally determined that exposure sessions in excess of one to two hours are superior to a series of shorter sessions.[25,26] In fact, short sessions of flooding, under 30 or 40 minutes, may result in increased anxiety. Consistent with the extinction theory, several studies have shown that during exposure, anxiety rises, peaks, then gradually diminishes. Edna Foa and Diane Chambless found this pattern with agoraphobics and with obsessive-compulsives. For the agoraphobics, SUDS ratings of anxiety peaked at about 45 minutes into the session before trailing off.[27] Had the sessions lasted only 45 minutes or less, the subjects would have been left in a state of heightened anxiety.

A second variation concerns the differential effectiveness of *in vivo* versus imaginal exposure. Although both forms have been found to be effective, most of the research shows the superiority of flooding *in vivo* in which the subject directly confronts the anxiety-provoking situation.[28]

With *in vivo* flooding, the person is taken directly to the situation that is feared. For example, with agoraphobia in which *in vivo* flooding is found quite effective, patients may be directed to leave their house or the therapist's office and begin walking for a specified time or distance. Often they are assisted or accompanied by a therapist. In some situations, this type of exposure can be done effectively with groups as well.[29] For some phobics, the anxiety and avoidance response may be so severe that they are initially unable to tolerate live exposure. In these cases, a few sessions of imaginal exposure might reduce their anxiety sufficiently to enable them to tolerate the live exposure.

A third procedure that appears to facilitate progress is self-directed practice between therapist-assisted flooding sessions. This addition to the more formal sessions increases the amount of exposure time and places patients in a practice situation that they personally control.[30] This element of having the persons themselves engage in the feared situation and direct their own efforts enhances their self-confidence as well.

Graduated Exposure

Another variant related to self-directed practice is *graduated exposure*, in which the subject confronts the feared situation until considerable anxiety is experienced. The patient then retrenches and later tries to increase the time spent in exposure. This graduated, self-directed exposure appears to be at least as effective as intense immersion in the situation and also offers the subject the sense of being more in control.[31] This form of graduated exposure, controlled by the subject, is quite similar to *in vivo* desensitization mentioned previously.

Response Prevention

Yet another variation of the exposure techniques is response prevention. Used with obsessive-compulsive disorders, response prevention entails preventing the obsessive-compulsive subject from engaging in his or her compulsive ritual while in the presence of the stimuli which typically generate the urge and the behavior.[32] For example, applied to an obsessive-compulsive hand washer who feels compelled to wash his hands each time he touches something with his bare hands, the therapist might encourage the person to touch a door knob, but refrain from hand washing, even though the urge is strong. This response prevention, like exposure in general, would result initially in intense anxiety over the urge to wash.

The anxiety generated from being exposed to the ritual-inducing stimulus (e.g., dirty door knob) eventually subsides as does the urge to perform the ritual. Response prevention and exposure are typically used together as a treatment package. However, many obsessive-compulsive disorders are exceedingly difficult to treat and these procedures are not universally successful when applied by themselves.[33,34] *Modeling*, another component of treatment, which was found to be highly successful with fears and phobias, appears to add significantly overall to treatment effectiveness.

Interoceptive Exposure

In Chapter 5, while discussing Barlow's theory of panic disorder, interoceptive cues were described as internal sensations that had become cues to elicit panic attacks. It was noted that many panic attacks that seemed to come out of the blue, were, in fact, cued by internal changes in physiological function, such as dizziness, change in heart rate, and the like. Exposing the panic-disordered person to these internal cues serves the same purpose as exposure to external panic-eliciting situations.

To expose persons to their panic-eliciting internal cues, several methods can be used. Persons whose panic might result from heart rate changes can be exposed by having them engage in some physical exercise, such as simply stepping up and down at a rapid pace, or running in place. Once they begin to feel symptoms, they then can either experience them until they no longer elicit an anxiety response or they can implement other anxiety control measures like relaxation or self-talk to inhibit the anxiety. Hyperventilation is another common process by which many panic attacks are initiated. Having the person rapidly breathe, as if they were blowing up a balloon, can stimulate numerous panic-related sensations, such as dizziness, tingling, lightheadedness, and weak knees. Spinning around in a swivel chair can also elicit the symptoms and serve as means to expose persons to their panic-eliciting cues. Such internal cue exposure can be very effective in eliminating these cues from eliciting anxiety attacks. Furthermore, they provide the person with an opportunity to practice using anxiety-coping procedures in a controlled and safe environment.

The Modeling Treatments

Observing others perform a behavior is one of the primary means by which we learn. As noted in Chapter 2, fears can be acquired vicariously by observing others undergo frightening or traumatic events. Conversely, fear can be reduced by modeling or observing someone else perform a feared act or interact with an anxiety-provoking object. Fear reduction by observing others perform a feared act appears to operate primarily through the process of vicarious extinction, similar to the effects seen in the exposure treatments. However, several other elements may be operating as well to contribute to the effectiveness of modeling. Through observing others, a person can obtain knowledge and information about the feared object and actually see what it is like. Furthermore, the observer can see how to enact the required fearless behavior that had been previously prevented by avoidance. As with the other fear and anxiety treatments, there are several variants of the modeling procedures and several factors that enhance their effectiveness. The modeling can be conducted in symbolic form or live.

In *symbolic modeling*, the model is shown on film or videotape. The observer (fearful person) simply views the film in which the model is depicted engaging in the feared actions. *Live modeling* proceeds the same way except that the modeling is done in person. Although symbolic modeling could be most economical in terms of time (not requiring another person to always be present), live modeling is generally considered more effective.[35]

Another dimension that facilitates the effectiveness of modeling is perceived similarity of the model; that is, the greater the similarity that fearful observers perceive between themselves and the model, the more they can identify with the model and, hence, the greater the fear reduction.

The use of multiple, as opposed to single, models also appears to enhance the overall effectiveness of modeling for fear reduction.[36] With several models demonstrating the feared behavior, there is greater likelihood that at least one of the models will be perceived as similar to the observer. Multiple models also show the observer that not just one person can do it but several can.

The model's manner of dealing with the feared situation also appears to make a difference. The most effective demeanor of the model is one in which initial apprehension is displayed. Then, the model progressively copes more and more effectively (less fearfully) with the situation. This use of a *coping model* has been shown to be superior to a *mastery model* in which the model demonstrates from the outset total control and no fearful behavior at all.[37] The use of a coping model may be more effective since the initial apprehension displayed and subsequent attempts to cope make the model appear more similar to the patient. Thus, the coping model is fearful just like the patient and is therefore perceived as more similar to the observer.

A variation in modeling procedure related to coping models is the use of graduated sequences. In *graduated modeling*, the modeled scenes are presented in a fashion similar to the anxiety hierarchy procedure from SD. Beginning with mildly anxiety-provoking scenes, successive scenes are graded to be progressively more and more threatening.[38]

For the most effective fear reduction, a combination of the above elements should be included in the procedure, including use of a live model similar to the subject who is shown to cope progressively with increasingly more threatening situations. However, in this type of modeling, the person is essentially a passive observer. Although such passive modeling has been shown to be effective in reducing fears and phobias, a more active form—*participant modeling*—is even more effective.[39]

Participant modeling involves direct interaction between the therapist, who can also serve as model, and the patient. It also involves direct exposure to the feared stimulus. As a general procedure, the model–therapist director demonstrates each step of the feared behavior, beginning with relatively simple situations. After each step is modeled, the therapist invites the subject to try it. If the subject is able to perform the task, the next step is demonstrated and the subject is then invited to try this second one, and so on. If the subject is not able to do it alone, the therapist might model the step again before inviting the subject to try. For example, for a snake phobic, the first step might be simply to enter a room with a caged, harmless snake. Then, with encouragement and support the subject may follow the lead of the therapist model and approach the cage, perhaps only a few steps at a time. Next, the therapist might open the cage, touch, pet, and eventually pick up the snake, inviting the subject to follow suit. The reader will probably note here that this procedure is similar to and combines elements of *in vivo* desensitization, graded exposure, and modeling, along with strong doses of support and encouragement to enable the subject to perform the feared act.

In addition to the above procedures, *performance aids* can be used to assist patients in approaching the feared situation. Using the snake phobic example, gloves might be used initially to encourage subjects to touch the snake. After the subject becomes comfortable touching the snake with gloves on, the performance aids are withdrawn and the subject is encouraged to use his or her bare hands.

Another procedure used to encourage performing the feared act is direct physical assistance by the therapist. Again using the snake example, this assistance could take the form of the subject's placing his or her hand on the therapist's hand who then touches the snake. Once this is accomplished, the therapist's hand is progressively withdrawn until the subject alone is touching the snake.

These forms of assistance to subjects are readily adaptable to the treatment of other disorders as well. For example, in treating an agoraphobic person fearful of entering a department store, the therapist or anyone who can provide comfort or a feeling of security could initially accompany the patient into the store. Then, after the person became reasonably comfortable with assistance, the helper could gradually increase the distance from the patient. Eventually, the assistant might wait outside while the person goes in alone, and so on.

All these active procedures are designed to get the fearful individual into contact with the feared object or situation and are enhanced by encouraging the person to practice on his or her own between treatment sessions.[40] It would appear to be important to the subject at one level to have successfully performed a previously feared behavior with the assistance of a therapist. The self-directed practice then takes patients a step closer to mastering their fears, panics, and anxiety. This success not only demonstrates that they can do it with assistance, but that they can also do it alone. This sense of mastery over a previously threatening situation is seen by some professionals as the central cognitive process that underlies behavior change. I will return shortly to this issue of underlying processes in fear and anxiety change.

Breathing Retraining

Doesn't everyone know how to breathe properly? Well, not everyone. Often, when people are tense, feel under stress, and are generally anxious, they *hyperventilate;* that is, they breathe too rapidly and too shallowly to promote a proper balance between carbon dioxide and oxygen throughout the body. One of the effects of this hyperventilation can be anxietylike symptoms that for some people trigger a panic attack.[41] For example, if you were intentionally to breathe rapidly as if you were blowing up a balloon, you might begin to feel dizzy, lightheaded, confused, have blurred vision, and feel tingling in your skin. These are normal reactions to hyperventilation and also symptoms of panic attacks. For some people, these feelings may frighten them enough to actually begin a panic attack.

To change this pattern of hyperventilation, a program of breathing retraining can be instituted. Measured, controlled breathing both prevents hyperventilation and promotes relaxation. The process of breathing retraining involves training persons to pace their breathing by focusing on a pattern of smooth, regular, and slow inhalation and expiration. Also instituted is deep breathing from the diaphragm as singers are trained to do. Rather than breathing by expanding the chest with each inhalation, the person is instructed to push the stomach out, which expands the diaphragmatic muscles at the base of the lungs. This process allows more oxygen to be taken in per breath.

Breathing retraining becomes a valuable technique for treating panic attacks. First, by preventing hyperventilation, it prevents some attacks themselves. As a relaxation procedure, slow, deep breathing can be instituted immediately when an attack begins. Using it early in an escalating attack can serve to abort the attack or to control its intensity and duration and thus can become a useful panic self-control technique. Breathing retraining has been found to be a highly successful panic treatment technique by itself for hyperventilators and is often used as part of comprehensive treatment programs, such as Barlow's *panic control treatment*.[42]

The Cognitive Restructuring Approaches

There are several related treatment methods that fall under the general classification of cognitive restructuring. All have a common aim of effecting change in a person's thinking or cognitive processes. The assumption underlying these approaches is that emotional disorders result, at least in part, from inappropriate, irrational, and self-defeating thoughts, concerns, or beliefs. We have all seen people who worry themselves sick and whose irrational focus on seemingly minor problems escalates them into intense anxiety and even full-blown panic attacks. Often, it is not the problem or the situation itself that causes an individual's problems; rather it is what the individual thinks about the situation that creates the anxiety and the associated avoidance. Depending on one's interpretation of an event, or what one thinks or says to oneself, the response may be one of fear and avoidance or of no fear and approach. In other words, how one thinks, in large part, determines how one feels and behaves. Therefore, treatment is directed toward altering thought processes that are related to the cause or maintenance of fear or anxiety responses.

As noted, there are several approaches that generally follow this cognitive model. For example, one of the first of these theorists was Albert Ellis who developed the procedure he termed *rational emotive therapy.*[43] Independently, Aaron Beck developed a similar approach, *cognitive therapy,* that focuses on changing irrational and illogical thoughts as a means of treating psychological difficulties.[44] The term, *cognitive restructuring,* came from the writings of Arnold Lazarus in which he described some cognitive approaches to behavior change as adjuncts to earlier behavior therapy procedures such as SD. More recently, Donald Meichenbaum, drawing in part from these other approaches, developed a cognitive restructuring procedure called *self-instructional training* (SIT).[46] Meichenbaum's SIT will now be described as a prototype of the cognitive restructuring approaches because it incorporates elements of the other cognitive approaches along with the other treatments described earlier. This procedure might best be seen as a general approach to treatment rather than as a specific technique.

Meichenbaum described *self-instructional training* as a three-phase therapy process: (1) providing information and assessment of the relation between thoughts and anxiety or fear response, (2) trying out new alternative ways of thinking which fit the person and the problem, and (3) using in actual practice new self-statements in the presence of the anxiety-provoking situation.

In Phase 1, individuals are provided with a conceptualization of their problem that enables them to realize the relation between thoughts, emotions, and behavior; that it is not really the situation that causes their fear, but what they think and say to themselves about the situation. For example, an agoraphobic person who becomes exceedingly anxious at the thought of being out alone may say, "What if I have a panic attack" or "What if I faint." This thinking, in turn, leads to anticipatory anxiety and to avoidance of going out.

The goal then of Phase 1 is to have subject realize this connection between thinking catastrophic thoughts and the self-defeating anxiety they elicit. Initially, this may be done by having persons simply imagine themselves in this situation and attend to the thoughts or self-statements that occur and the resulting anxiety. Also, homework assignments may be given, such as having patients monitor and record thoughts and feelings they experience between sessions and note the relationship between them. Once subjects are able to see clearly the connection between their thinking processes and how they affect behavior, the next phase can be introduced.

Phase 2 involves developing and testing new things to do and to think that can prevent and/or counter the fear and anxiety responses. These new things would include learning relaxation techniques that could be used to help individuals prepare for and cope with an anxiety-provoking situation. Also, new self-statements and thoughts about situations could be tried and rehearsed. Here, Meichenbaum introduced another procedure that he called *stress-inoculation training*. In stress inoculation, the patients develop statements to say to themselves prior to meeting the stressor, such as "No negative thoughts, worry won't help," "Just think about what you have to do." Then, when actually in the situation, another set of self-statements can be used to keep patients on task and use coping skills: "Take this one step at a time," "Take a deep breath and begin relaxing," "You can do it, just hang on." These self-statements are designed to keep the patients' on task and to remind them what to do. As the fear begins to develop, the patient then might say, "It is only fear; it won't really hurt me," "Let it come but keep it manageable."

Once the fear has passed, patients then need to reinforce themselves for having tolerated it and gotten through it: "You did it," "It worked." The development of these self-statements gives patients something constructive to do to cope with fear-provoking situations. The self-statements are then used to counter and challenge negative thoughts that emerge into patients' thinking, and to help them with the task of working to reduce the response, rather than letting the anxiety-provoking thoughts take over.

Phase 3 of SIT can begin once a person has developed and tried out a series of new self-statements and coping skills. Phase 3 is the actual use of these skills in feared situations. Here the full package of new skills, thinking, self-statements, and relaxation is put to use to enable the person to begin tolerating previously feared situations. Other procedures might also be enlisted to facilitate this process. For example, Meichenbaum would encourage subjects to use a variant of SD, such as that described by Goldfried in which anxiety hierarchy scenes are visualized with the person coping with and attempting to reduce the felt anxiety. These scenes might actually involve the person visualizing himself or herself being in the situation, making coping self-statements, and being able to tolerate it. In other words, the procedure combines elements of SD and covert or imaginal self-modeling, along with changes in self-statements.

Self-instructional training may then be seen as a treatment package incorporating elements and adaptations of other fear-reduction methods. These methods are used to assist fearful persons to change self-defeating thoughts and to enable them to tolerate and cope with being in the presence of the feared situation until the fear diminishes.

Throughout this chapter, the reader will have noticed that the several treatment methods described progressed from a relatively structured set of procedures (systematic desensitization and symbolic modeling) to more comprehensive and inclusive treatment packages, such as participant modeling and cognitive restructuring. This trend toward incorporating a broad assortment of methods reflects what therapists do clinically. They draw upon established procedures and adapt them to the specific needs of their patients. What fits for some patients or problems may not fit others. This integration of the several treatments in practice will be further illustrated in the next chapter in which applications to specific anxiety disorders are described.

Another point that readers might have noticed is that the various anxiety-treatment procedures described were in some cases quite different or appeared even opposite. For example, the standard SD procedure attempts to insulate the person from feeling too much anxiety, whereas flooding attempts to *create* anxiety. Yet each of these techniques boasts substantial research support attesting to its effectiveness in reducing anxiety disorders. How do these seemingly divergent treatment techniques all produce significant reductions in fear and anxiety? Do they each operate through different mechanisms or is there some process common to all that can explain their effectiveness? In the following section, I will present one theoretical position that attempts to account for the behavior change seen in all these techniques.

Self-Efficacy Theory

Albert Bandura of Stanford University presented a unifying theory of behavior change that explains the effectiveness of the various treatment procedures. According to Bandura, behavior change derives from a common cognitive process which essentially is the individual's personal belief that he or she can perform a desired but feared behavior, such as taking a trip on an airplane. This belief, which is termed an *efficacy expectation*, reflects the extent to which an individual holds the expectation that he or she can perform a given act successfully. The more positive one's efficacy expectation, the greater the probability that one will be able to perform. Of course, actual performance also depends on the extent to which the person wants to perform an act and expects that the outcome will be worth the effort.

With respect to fear behavior, a person phobic of enclosed places like elevators would be expected to have low *self-efficacy* concerning his or her ability to enter an elevator and allow the doors to close. Accordingly, the probability of that person's actually entering an elevator would be correspondingly low.

According to Bandura, the task of the several fear-reducing treatments is to increase the fearful person's sense of self-efficacy which, in turn, will increase the probability that the person will perform the anxiety-provoking behavior. This sense of self-efficacy is derived from various sources. Bandura attributed the effectiveness of the seemingly different treatments to the fact that they all contribute to enhancing the fearful person's sense of self-efficacy. Although each of the techniques described previously is somewhat effective, some are more effective than others. Bandura believed that this differential effectiveness is due to differences in the extent to which the techniques enhance an individual's self-efficacy. Thus, Bandura grouped the various techniques according to the source through which each operates to provide efficacy expectations. The sources are: performance accomplishments, vicarious experiences, verbal persuasion, and emotional arousal.

Performance Accomplishments

The performance-based procedures in which the fearful person actively interacts with the feared situation are the most effective treatment procedures. The techniques used include live exposure, participant modeling, and self-directed practice.[47] Their effectiveness is believed to be a result of the fact that once a step is actually accomplished, the individual is able to see clearly what he or she has achieved. The self-observation of personal accomplishment is the most dependable source of efficacy expectations. They are based on one's personal experience. Having successfully approached and touched a snake, even with aid and support, or having tolerated a session of intense exposure at a shopping mall by an agoraphobic, is very strong evidence that it can be done again. This direct accomplishment strongly enhances one's self-efficacy which, in turn, increases the probability that next time one will be able to go even further in combating one's fear.

Vicarious Experiences

A second source of efficacy information is provided by observing others perform a feared act in live or symbolic modeling. Although seen by themselves as providing less clear evidence that the observer can perform similarly, these vicarious experiences can enhance efficacy expectations. Observing multiple models who gradually, but with persistence, overcome their hesitations and are able to perform the feared act, can create expectations in the observer that he or she can also perform the act.

Verbal Persuasion

Techniques that involve verbal persuasion, such as suggestion, exhortation, or attempts to verbally convince a person that he or she can perform a feared act, are seen as relatively weak sources of self-efficacy enhancement. Although such efforts might encourage a person to try to perform the behavior, by themselves they do little to help a person overcome intense fear. Recall that a defining characteristic of phobia was that individuals could not be talked out of their fears.

However, verbal methods might be sufficient to convince a person to make an initial attempt to overcome a particular fear. If this initial attempt results in some degree of success, the self-efficacy should be increased and should facilitate further efforts. However, if the attempt meets with negative consequences, the small amount of self-efficacy provided verbally is not likely to maintain persistent efforts. A common example of this is seen in persons who are fearful of dentistry. Often a fearful person will be persuaded by his or her spouse to make a dental appointment after years of avoidance. If the dentist is not cognizant of the extent of the person's fear or is not knowledgeable in fear treatment, a negative experience may well result. The person is unlikely to return for some time. On the other hand, if the experience with the dentist is positive and nontraumatic and the person is able to tolerate it, his or her self-efficacy would be greatly enhanced and a return visit would be likely. However, the major source of efficacy expectation here is from the fearful person's actual performance accomplishment, although the persuasion was important in getting the person into the situation to allow the accomplishment.

Emotional Arousal

The final source of efficacy expectations suggested by Bandura is how people sense themselves reacting physiologically. When confronted with a potentially threatening situation, the degree of fear and avoidance behavior that is shown may be partly a function of one's perception of the physical arousal that is experienced. If our heart races, we are likely to label ourselves as fearful. On the other hand, if we find we do not become unduly physically aroused, we are less likely to label ourselves fearful. Thus, the cues from our internal state provide information concerning whether or not we expect to be able to tolerate the situation. Treatment techniques that focus on reducing physical arousal then can contribute to one's sense of self-efficacy. These include relaxation-based procedures, such as systematic desensitization, biofeedback, and breathing retraining, as well as drug treatments which reduce the physical arousal. (The use of drugs in anxiety reduction will be described in Chapter 10.)

According to Bandura, these treatments provide some information that enhances efficacy expectations. Through lowered arousal, people who are fearful come to expect less fearful behavior in themselves which then allows them to approach or tolerate the feared situation. However, as with the method of verbal persuasion, the lasting effects of decreased arousal are obtained by enabling the person to enter the feared situation and ultimately to experience performance accomplishment.

In summary, Bandura's theory proposes self-efficacy as the common cognitive mechanism to explain the effectiveness of the several treatments. Any source of information that contributes to enhancing a person's expectations for success will contribute to overcoming fearful avoidance behavior.

REFERENCES

1. Albert Bandura, Edward Blanchard, and B. Ritter, "Relative Efficacy of Desensitization and Modeling Approaches for Inducing Behavioral, Affective, and Attitudinal Changes," *Journal of Personality and Social Psychology* 13 (1969): 173–199.
2. Stanley Rachman and Ray Hodgson, *Obsessions and Compulsions* (Englewood Cliffs, N.J.: Prentice-Hall, 1980).
3. Ibid.
4. Joseph Wolpe, *Psychotherapy by Reciprocal Inhibition* (Stanford, Cal.: Stanford University Press, 1958).
5. Ibid., 17.
6. Ibid.
7. Edmund Jacobson, *Progressive Relaxation* (Chicago: University of Chicago Press, 1938).
8. Douglas Bernstein and Thomas Borkovec, *Progressive Relaxation Training: A Manual for the Helping Professions* (Champaign, Ill.: Research Press, 1974).
9. Joseph Wolpe and Arnold Lazarus, *Behavior Therapy Techniques: A Guide to Treatment of the Neuroses* (Oxford, England: Pergamon Press, 1966).
10. Joseph Wolpe, *The Practice of Behavior Therapy* (Oxford, England: Pergamon, 1973).
11. Arnold Lazarus, "Group Therapy of Phobic Disorders by Systematic Desensitization," *Journal of Abnormal and Social Psychology* 63 (1973): 504–510.
12. Kenneth Ihli and Warren Garlington, "A Comparison of Group versus Individual Desensitization of Test Anxiety," *Behaviour Research and Therapy* 7 (1969): 207–210.
13. Gordon Paul and Donald Shannon, "Treatment of Anxiety through Systematic Desensitization in Therapy Groups," *Journal of Abnormal Psychology* 71 (1966): 124–135.
14. David Sue, "The Effect of Duration of Exposure on Systematic Desensitization and Extinction," *Behaviour Research and Therapy* 13 (1975): 55–60.
15. Stanley J. Rachman, "Studies in Desensitization II: Flooding," *Behaviour Research and Therapy* 4 (1966): 1–6.
16. Peter Lang, Barbara Melamed, and I. Hart, "A Psychophysiological Analysis of Fear Modification Using an Automated Desensitization Procedure," *Journal of Abnormal Psychology* 76 (1970): 220–234.

17. B. Migler and Joseph Wolpe, "Automated Desensitization: A Case Report," *Behaviour Research and Therapy* 5 (1967): 133.
18. L. Donner and B. G. Guerney, "Automated Group Desensitization for Test Anxiety," *Behaviour Research and Therapy* 7 (1969), 1–13.
19. Marvin Goldfried, "Systematic Desensitization as Training in Self-Control," *Journal of Consulting and Clinical Psychology* 37 (1971): 228–234.
20. Wolpe, *The Practice of Behavior Therapy.*
21. Zol Garfield, P. L. Darwin, B. A. Singer, and J. McBreaty, "Effect of 'In Vivo' Training on Experimental Desensitization of a Phobia," *Psychological Reports* 20 (1967): 515–519.
22. K. D. O'Leary and G. T. Wilson, *Behavior Therapy: Application and Outcome,* (Englewood Cliffs, N.J.: Prentice-Hall, 1975).
23. M. Girodo, "Yoga Meditation and Flooding in Treatment of Anxiety Neurosis," *Journal of Behavior Therapy and Experimental Psychiatry* 5 (1974): 157–160.
24. Rachman and Hodgson, *Obsessions and Compulsions.*
25. Stanley Rachman and G. T. Wilson, *The Effects of Psychological Therapy,* 2nd ed. (Oxford, England: Pergamon Press, 1980).
26. Richard Stern and Isaac Marks, "Brief and Prolonged Flooding: A Comparison in Agoraphobic Patients," *Archives of General Psychiatry* 28 (1973): 270–276.
27. Edna Foa and Diane Chambless, "Habituation of Subjective Anxiety during Flooding in Imagery," *Behaviour Research and Therapy* 16 (1978): 391–399.
28. Stern and Marks, "Brief and Prolonged Flooding."
29. Julian Hafner and Isaac Marks, "Exposure *In Vivo* of Agoraphobics: Contributions of Diazepam, Group Exposure and Anxiety Evocation, *Psychological Medicine* 6 (1976): 71–88.
30. A. Mathews, J. Teasdale, M. Munby, D. Johnston, and P. Shaw, "A Home Based Treatment Program for Agoraphobia," *Behavior Therapy* 8 (1977): 915–924.
31. Paul Emmelkamp, *Phobic and Obsessive-Compulsive Disorders* (New York: Plenum Press, 1982).
32. Rachman and Hodgson, *Obsessions and Compulsions.*
33. Ibid.
34. Paul Emmelkamp and H. Wessels, "Flooding in Imagination vs. Flooding *In Vivo*: A Comparison with Agoraphobics," *Behaviour Research and Therapy* 13 (1975): 7–16.
35. Albert Bandura, *Principles of Behavior Modification* (New York: Holt, 1969).
36. Albert Bandura and Francis Menlove, "Factors Determining Vicarious Extinction of Avoidance Behavior through Symbolic Modeling," *Journal of Personality and Social Psychology* 8 (1968): 99–108.
37. Alan Kazdin, "The Affect of Model Identity and Fear-Relevant Similarity on Covert Modeling," *Behavior Therapy* 5 (1974): 624–635.
38. Bandura, *Principles of Behavior Modification.*

39. Albert Bandura, *Social Learning Theory* (Englewood Cliffs, N.J.: Prentice-Hall, 1977).

40. Ibid.

41. David Barlow, *Anxiety and Its Disorders* (New York: Guilford Press, 1988).

42. David Barlow and Mischelle Craske, *Mastery of Your Anxiety and Panic* (Albany, N.Y.: Greywind Publications, 1989).

43. Albert Ellis, *Reason and Emotion in Psychotherapy* (New York: Lyle Stuart, 1962).

44. Aaron Beck, *Cognitive Therapy and the Emotional Disorders* (New York: International Universities Press, 1976).

45. Arnold Lazarus, *Behavior Therapy and Beyond* (New York: McGraw-Hill, 1971).

46. Donald Meichenbaum, *Cognitive-Behavior Modification: An Integrative Approach* (New York: Plenum Press, 1977).

47. Bandura, *Social Learning Theory*.

CHAPTER 9

Anxiety Disorders Treatment Programs

The reduction procedures for fear and anxiety described in the previous chapter are now applied as treatments to specific anxiety disorders. As is most often the case in clinical practice, several procedures are used with the same individual in order to capitalize on the most effective elements of each and to adapt the treatment to the specific characteristics and needs of the individual client. The cases that follow were selected to illustrate how the various procedures can be adapted effectively and combined into comprehensive individualized treatment programs.

TREATMENT OF SIMPLE PHOBIAS

A Dental Phobia

This case study, which was conducted by Douglas Bernstein and myself, illustrates the use of a combination of three treatment procedures to assist the subject in overcoming a long-standing fear and avoidance of dental treatment.[1]

The subject, Mrs. W., was a 37-year-old woman who had avoided dentistry for the previous six years. However, several months prior to this treatment, she had attempted an appointment to have her teeth cleaned but was unable to complete it because of a severe anxiety reaction. When seated in the dental chair, she experienced profuse sweating, shortness of breath, gagging, weakness in her knees, muscular tension, and nausea. Her reaction was so intense that despite the administration of nitrous oxide she was unable to tolerate having her teeth cleaned.

Mrs. W.'s fear reaction went far beyond her being in the dental office: she was unable to call for an appointment either for herself or for her children. Her husband not only had to take the children to their appointments but also had to call to set up her fear-treatment appointment. Furthermore, if at anytime the subject of dentistry was brought up, it would later stimulate dreams in which Mrs. W. saw her teeth shattered and then fall out. Although Mrs. W. knew that her reaction was irrational, she was totally unable to control it. Clearly, she met the criteria for phobia.

Prior to the beginning of the fear treatment, a series of assessments were completed to evaluate Mrs. W.'s fear reaction and later to provide a baseline against which to compare treatment effectiveness. The assessment was conducted in a dental office but she was told that no actual treatment would take place. While she was sitting in the dental chair, the cognitive component of state anxiety was assessed with an instrument called the *Anxiety Differential*, which provided a measure of her current anxiety state. Three measurements of her physiological arousal were taken with the Palmar Sweat Index (PSI): (1) as she entered the dental operatory, (2) before receiving an anesthetic injection (she refused to have it), and (3) at the end of the assessment session. (The PSI is a measure of the number of open sweat pores in a designated area of the finger.) These assessment measures were taken again after treatment.

Following the assessment, the treatment consisted of four components: (1) training in muscle relaxation, (2) symbolic modeling, (3) graduated exposure to dental stimuli presented on video tape, and (4) self-paced live exposure practice in which she went to the dental office, and practiced relaxing while being exposed to the sights, sounds, and smells of dentistry.

This sequence of treatments was planned for Mrs. W. to gradually reintroduce her to dentistry. While providing her with relaxation as a coping skill, she also obtained information about how dentistry proceeds without her receiving negative direct experiences. And through modeling, she could observe how several other people (models) coped with their treatment. After viewing several coping models receive treatment, her anxiety was lessened. Then the graduated exposure, also on video tape, allowed her to observe in a safe manner elements of dental treatment while she practiced remaining relaxed. Finally, on her own, she scheduled two sessions in which she went to the dental office to practice these skills. The first time she was instructed simply to sit in the waiting room, attend to the sounds and sights of dentistry, and to practice coping with them. Once this step was mastered, her next appointment involved her going into the dental operatory, sitting and relaxing in the dental chair, being exposed to the various instruments (e.g., the drill), but without being actually treated. This live exposure, coupled with the previous information, allowed an informed, first-hand experience with dentistry that was nontraumatic. By introducing the dental stimuli slowly and progressively, she was able to tolerate each succeeding step. The entire procedure took only 3.5 hours of my professional time.

Following the successful completion of this program, Mrs. W. scheduled a badly needed treatment appointment. At this appointment, her fear responses were again evaluated. The posttreatment assessment was objectively more stressful than the pretreatment one since she was to have three teeth filled. In spite of the added stress of actual dental treatment, her state anxiety score decreased significantly and her PSI showed a reversal of the pretreatment pattern. On the first assessment, the PSI pattern showed progressively more sweating throughout the appointment. On the second session during treatment, the pattern was one of continuously decreasing sweating. Perhaps the most impressive evidence of treatment effectiveness was the fact that during the 12 months following treatment, Mrs. W. had five additional appointments at which she had a total of eight fillings, a root canal, a replaced crown, a repair of a fractured tooth, and her teeth cleaned.

A Thunderstorm Phobia

This case of a longstanding thunderstorm phobia was described by Lars-Goran Öst from the University of Uppsala in Sweden.[2]

> The patient was a 77-year-old Swedish woman who had been phobic since childhood. Each spring, she would begin worrying about possible summer thunderstorms. She routinely avoided listening to weather forecasts since knowledge of impending storms would increase her anxiety. During a storm she experienced chest pains, trembling, and felt panicky. She would crawl into places in her house and bury her face in a pillow so she could not see the storm.

The treatment for this case included a two-stage process involving relaxation training, followed by a variant of systematic desensitization referred to by Öst as "self-administered desensitization."

Prior to treatment, a series of four assessment sessions were conducted in which fear reactions were measured. Since thunderstorms do not occur on demand, Öst constructed a laboratory simulation of a storm. He played a tape recording of actual thunder that was synchronized with a series of slides depicting approaching storm clouds with lightning. Also flashing lights were used to increase the realism of the lightning.

While experiencing these sights and sounds, several fear measures were taken: self-report measures included a thunder-and-lightning phobia scale and a 0–10-point rating of degree of anxiety experienced during the test. Also, heart rate and respiration were measured throughout the simulated storm session.

After these initial fear measures were taken, the client was given five sessions of relaxation training with measurements taken during each session. The self-administered desensitization was then introduced for an additional eight sessions. This procedure consisted first of the client listening to a tape recording of her favorite music while practicing relaxation for four sessions. Then, for four more sessions, the client listened to the tape of thunderstorms while trying to maintain relaxation. If she became too anxious, she could turn the tape off and relax again. Then the process could be repeated until she could listen to the tape all the way through without undue anxiety. Evaluation of treatment effects showed progressive decreases in each of the fear measures. Most of the reduction in the fear measures occurred by the end of the relaxation phase. The self-rated anxiety went from 8 during baseline to 4 during relaxation and to 3 by the end of the self-administered desensitization. Her heart rate showed a decrease from an average of 175.6 beats per minute (BPM) to 69.7 BPM at the end of treatment.

During the nine months following treatment, this client reported that, for the first time in decades, she was able to enjoy a summer stay in Italy even though she had encountered several thunderstorms and that she no longer worried so much over the coming of summer storms.

Blood and Injury Phobia

Cohn, Kron, and Brady described an interesting treatment approach to relieve a 28-year-old man of his longstanding phobia of blood and injury.[3]

> Their patient was a premedical student with a master's degree in chemistry who had his fear since he was four years of age. At the sight of blood or injuries to others he reliably became light-headed and would faint if he did not quickly lie down. This reaction of course kept him from being a viable candidate for medical school.

Before treatment began, an assessment session was conducted to fully evaluate his physiological reactions. Recall that blood-injury phobics show a response pattern quite different from other phobics; they have a drop in blood pressure and heart rate that often results in fainting.

The assessment consisted of attaching the subject to an electrocardiograph to monitor his heart rate. He was then shown a series of slides of mutilated bodies along with a control slide of a cartoon. The slides were shown for varying lengths of time to observe how his heart rate changed. At exposures greater than 60 seconds, he reported feeling light-headed and his heart rate dropped from its normal rate of about 86 BPM to as low as 47 BPM. After 75 seconds, it dropped to 30 BPM, he fainted, then it rose to over 100.

The initial treatment consisted of a variant of systematic desensitization. He was asked to lie down on a couch and relax. Then, while relaxed, he was shown brief glimpses of the mutilation slides that he could turn off if he became light-headed. After a session of this treatment, he was able to extend the length of time he could view the slides, but only by a few seconds.

In the next session, the researchers tried something different. They decided to use a response that would be incompatible with fear but that would keep the blood pressure up. Anger appeared to be such a response. Accordingly, with the subject's help, they identified several situations that aroused the subject to anger. These anger-arousing situations included mention of his father, an argument with his wife, and his college advisor. Then, while viewing the phobic slides, the therapists, playing the role of antagonists, aroused the subject to anger. Viewing the slides while angry was no problem. The patient was able to do so immediately for periods of as long as 20 minutes and to maintain his heart rate within the normal range of 70 to 90 BPM.

Following this successful session, he was given a homework assignment to practice on his own. He received a medical textbook with pictures of mutilated bodies, was asked to look at horror movies, and to read books that had previously caused him to faint. He was to maintain his anger while participating in these tasks for several 30-minute practice sessions per week.

After four weeks of this successful practice, he gave up the anger and pictures and became a volunteer worker in the emergency room of a general hospital. After six months, he had not fainted once, despite his extensive exposure to the previously faint-producing situations.

The authors of this report suggested that the treatment was probably successful on account of two processes. First, by being angry, the patient did not identify so closely with the injured person. Second, the anger kept the patient's blood pressure and heart rate elevated, which prevented him from fainting long enough to allow himself to become habituated to the gory scenes.

A Life-Threatening Case of Claustrophobia

A life-saving treatment of claustrophobia was conducted by Elizabeth Klonoff and Jeffrey Janata from Case Western Reserve University.[4]

> Their patient, a 43-year-old woman, had endocrinologic signs suggestive of a pituitary gland tumor. To verify and precisely locate the tumor so they could decide whether surgery was required and/or possible, they needed to obtain a brain image using a highly sophisticated brain-scanning procedure called Magnetic Resonance Imaging (MRI). Unfortunately, the apparatus that housed the MRI device required that the person's head be encased in a metal cylinder for time periods of between 20 and 45 minutes, a near impossible task for a claustrophobic person. On a first attempt, she was unable to stay in long enough for a useable scan. It became clear that a phobia treatment program would have to be initiated.

The phobia treatment consisted of *in vivo* desensitization and began with teaching the patient how to relax deeply. Then, she was instructed to practice relaxing at home with her head inside of a small box. After she was able to do this, she was brought back to the radiology laboratory and helped to relax while lying on the MRI machine without being slid into the apparatus. As she accomplished this relaxation, she was slowly but progressively moved into the apparatus, but at a pace she chose and at which she was able to maintain her relaxation. She was then able to remain in the machine for 20 minutes, which was long enough to obtain a successful image of the tumor. This relatively simple treatment took only four treatment sessions to accomplish.

Scriptophobia

The treatment of scriptophobia to be described is one of three such cases treated by Biran, Augusto, and Wilson.[5] (This case history was included in the description of social phobias presented in Chapter 4.)

> This scriptophobic patient was 37 years old at the time of treatment and had been phobic of writing in public since she was 16 years old. Due to her fear, she was unable to participate in any activity that required her to write in public, such as purchasing items with checks or bank cards, or voting. Although she was working part-time as a typist, her work was impaired due to her phobia. She was less anxious, however, when in the presence of a trusted family member or when out of direct public view.
>
> When in a situation requiring writing she experienced palpitations, shortness of breath, sweating, and shakiness, particularly of the hands. She avoided such situations over her concern that others would see her shake and look anxious. She feared that they would wonder what was wrong with her.
>
> Assessment of her phobia included several cognitive self-report and behavioral measures. Before and after treatment she was given the Fear of Negative Evaluation Scale, which showed her to be highly anxious over others' evaluation of her. The Rathus Assertiveness Scale indicated that she was quite unassertive and would not stick up for her rights.

A behavioral avoidance test was constructed that included a graded series of 13 tasks to be performed. Easier tasks included: filling out forms in the therapy room with the therapist observing and filling out forms alone in a hallway waiting area. More difficult tasks included: purchasing items at a store with a check, a credit card, and with travelers' checks. The BAT score was the number out of 13 of these situations she was able to perform. During the BAT, she also gave a subjective rating of her anxiety on a scale from 0 to 10.

She received five separate assessments: (1) pretreatment, (2) after treatment 1, (3) after treatment 2, (4) at 1-month follow-up, and (5) at 9-months follow-up. By this procedure, the therapist could separately evaluate effects of each of the two treatment procedures.

Since scriptophobia involves both a strong cognitive component (anticipatory anxiety and worry over social evaluation) and a behavioral component (avoidance of writing in public), the therapists felt that treatments should be chosen to focus specifically on these two areas. The first treatment was cognitive restructuring. As described in Chapter 8, cognitive restructuring involves explaining to the subject that it is not the situation *per se* that causes her anxiety, but rather what she thought about it. She then observed her own thinking to see how her thoughts and self-statements initiated her anxiety. Then, more realistic, nonanxiety-producing thoughts were identified and practiced to replace the negative thoughts. These were practiced in her imagination and in role-playing with the therapist. She then was encouraged to practice on her own between treatment sessions.

Following five sessions of cognitive restructuring, the BAT was readministered. There was essentially no change in the number of tasks she could perform; four on both occasions. Her subjectively rated anxiety while performing the BAT was also unchanged. The procedure of cognitive restructuring had not worked.

At this point, five sessions of graded *in vivo* exposure treatment were initiated. The situations worked on were those from the BAT. However, performance at each task level was assisted by the therapist. For example, for purchasing items from a store using a checkbook, initially the therapist was present, which made it easier. As the client was able to accomplish this task, the therapist then moved further and further away while the client wrote the checks. She was eventually able to write them totally on her own.

After five sessions of this therapist-assisted exposure, the subject was reassessed on the BAT and was now able to perform all 13 tasks. Her subjective anxiety during these tasks dropped from a pretreatment average of 4 to an average of 1. One month following treatment, she was still able to complete all 13 tasks and her subjective anxiety was virtually nonexistent. However, the assessment nine months later showed conflicting results. Although she was still able to perform all 13 BAT tasks, her subjective anxiety had returned almost to her pretreatment level. Despite the return of some of the subjective anxiety, this client was able to maintain her behavioral gains. She became employed full-time, was able to shop with checks and credit cards, and to endorse checks at the bank, none of which she was able to perform prior to treatment.

The results of this case were generally consistent with the other two reported in this series of case studies. It thus appeared that the graded exposure treatment was most effective in reducing the behavioral-avoidance component of social phobia. The cognitive restructuring appeared to have minimal effect. Also, at one month posttreatment, all clients showed significant drops in subjective anxiety, but, at nine months, the disorder had returned to near pretreatment levels.

TREATMENT OF PANIC AND AGORAPHOBIA

Panic Disorder with Breathing Retraining

Ronald Rapee from the University of New South Wales, Australia, described one of the earliest examples of panic disorder that was treated with breathing retraining.[6] His client Ann, a 23-year-old woman, experienced approximately one panic attack per day, each lasting an average of one hour. These attacks had no apparent external cause; they seemed to come out of the blue. During the attacks she experienced the full range of panic symptoms, including palpitations, choking, lump in the throat, dizziness, and the like. Between attacks, she experienced general anxiety, depersonalization, and chronic chest pain. She was not taking any medications but required wine to get to sleep at night.

Rapee's treatment program consisted of three main aspects: (1) to inform Ann of how hyperventilation can cause the symptoms she experienced, (2) to have her increase her attention to her breathing pattern in the event that it were the cause of the symptoms, and (3) to provide her with training in breathing control.

To begin, Rapee asked Ann to hyperventilate intentionally for a period of 90 seconds. She noted that the symptoms she experienced in this exercise were very similar to those experienced during a panic attack. The treatment then consisted of having Ann learn to breathe by expanding her diaphragm and concentrating on bringing her breathing into a steady regular rhythm. Once this was accomplished, she was helped to slow her breathing down to a rate of 7 to 8 BPM. She was instructed to practice this two times each day for periods of 10 minutes. Finally, she was encouraged to use this new breathing pattern as a relaxant to ward off impending panic attacks as soon as she sensed one coming on.

For three weeks prior to beginning the treatment, Ann had kept daily records of her panic attacks. During this baseline period of 21 days, she had 22 attacks. During the three weeks following treatment, she had only two attacks, and these were quite mild because she was able to keep them under control. At 6-month follow-up, she was panic free.

Although all cases of panic disorder are neither as easily nor as quickly resolved as was Ann's, many can be. Such cases are particularly treatable if they stem specifically from hyperventilation and if techniques such as deep, diaphragmatic breathing work well for the patients. The following case history illustrates how a relatively modest success at controlling a panic attack can snowball into a rapid and complete recovery.

Eldon was a 61-year-old retired government employee who took early medical retirement because of a severe heart condition that ultimately required bypass surgery. Eldon had been an anxious person most of his life, but the recurrent panic attacks and resultant behavioral restriction had been progressively increasing over the past couple of years. At the time he sought treatment on referral from his cardiologist, Eldon was reluctant to drive if traffic was heavy and he would walk but a short distance from his home, even with the encouragement and insistence of his wife. He feared that, while out, he might have a panic attack, which he feared even more than having another heart attack. He stated that he did not fear heart attacks because he believed that doctors could treat those. Further, he stated that he did not fear death because he had already died once from his heart attack and felt that it was not so bad. It was living with panic that he feared because there was nothing he could do for the panics. He had virtually no self-efficacy with respect to dealing with a panic attack. He felt there was nothing he or his doctors could do.

Given this belief in the patient's inability to control an attack, the first line of treatment was directed at enhancing his self-efficacy on this count. The first step was to test the effects on Eldon of a slowed and deeper breathing pattern, with training in diaphragmatic breathing. Immediately, he felt relaxed. After discussing how he should monitor his breathing periodically throughout the day, Eldon was advised that if he felt a panic attack coming on, he was immediately to enter into this deep breathing and focus intently on relaxing. At the same time, he was given an article to read about the concept of self-efficacy and its importance for overcoming fear and avoidance behavior. Within a couple of days, Eldon ventured into a department store and, while waiting in line, began to have a panic attack. His first impulse was to leave. Then, he recalled the deep-breathing routine we had rehearsed, instituted it immediately, and found that the attack subsided to a manageable level. This experience at controlling an attack seemed to be all Eldon needed to restore his self-confidence. He now had a means to control the panic; he knew he could stop an attack. From this point on, he tried driving on the freeway again with great success for the first time in some months. He began taking long walks again which made him feel better and sleep better. With just these three treatment sessions, Eldon was again able to walk, travel, and visit with friends and family, all of which had been his stated goals at the initial meeting.

Like Rapee's case, Eldon's history was presented to illustrate how such treatments can work to restore pleasure and mobility to people's lives, with a minimum of time and effort in some instances. Unfortunately, other cases of panic disorder become more advanced to where agoraphobic avoidance has persisted for some time and has greatly restricted the patient to the point of being housebound. The following treatment program illustrates how these cases can be treated.

Housebound Agoraphobia

Agoraphobia can deprive its victims of most every aspect of life outside the home, leaving many housebound and totally dependent on "safe" others for excursions beyond the front door. In many cases, the fear is so great that the person is unable to come to clinics for treatment. In light of this difficulty, the program to be described took the treatment to the clients. In this novel and successful series of case studies, the clients were given a self-help treatment manual while the therapists served primarily as consultants and advisors.[7]

The patients in this treatment study were 12 married women whose agoraphobia had persisted from 1.5 to 20 years with an average of 9.3 years. All were disabled to the extent that they were unable to leave home alone to visit neighbors or to shop.

Prior to introducing the treatment programs, there was a 3-

week period of baseline assessment. The measures included a self-rating of symptom severity, ranging from 1, which indicated very little restriction, to 5, which indicated severe incapacitation. The average pretreatment rating was 4. Additionally, all patients kept diaries in which they recorded daily the amount of time they spent outside the home. Before treatment, this time period averaged 5 hours per week.

A third measure to evaluate treatment effectiveness was taken from a graded hierarchy of situations constructed during the baseline phase. With the aid of the therapist, 14 situations for each patient were listed as goals toward which they would work. The number of these goals the subject was able to accomplish was taken as a behavioral measure of treatment effectiveness. Low hierarchy goals included such things as walking alone to a friend's house or walking to a local bus stop. More difficult situations were walking to a local shop and taking a short bus ride. Items at the top of the list included taking a bus trip to a nearby town and visiting a social club. The patients were tested at three points to see how many of the 14 situations they could complete. They were tested during the baseline period, after four weeks of treatment practice, and six months following treatment.

After baseline evaluation, the therapist met with each patient and her husband at their home. At this meeting, they went over the detailed treatment manual and discussed procedures for implementing a graded exposure practice program. The manual described how to begin an exposure treatment program by setting up short treatment goals, allowing oneself to be exposed to a situation until the anxiety subsided and then going on to a more difficult goal.

An important ingredient in this program was that the spouse had to be totally involved in the treatment process. The husband and wife had to work together to plan the specific treatment steps and to carry them out. The husband was also given a manual to assist him in helping his wife. He had to participate in each of the one-hour per day practice sessions and to record the time spent and work accomplished.

The therapist served primarily as an advisor through the four weeks of the program. His role was to assist the husband and wife in setting practice goals, provide advice and support, and answer questions concerning the manual and the program. He was present only at the first practice session, but met with the couple a total of eight times over the four weeks to help them work through the program.

Following the 4 weeks of the actual treatment portion of the study, 11 of the 12 women had been able to enter at least one situation from their hierarchy that they had not been able to tolerate during the pretreatment assessment. Also, their self-rated severity of symptoms had declined to an average of 2.8, and the amount of time spent outside the home had more than doubled to an average of 11 hours by the end of the 4-week program.

At the 6-month follow-up assessment, these gains were either maintained or had increased. Although the time out of the home remained at about 11 hours per week, the severity rating had further decreased to 2.3, a level indicating no significant restriction because of a recurrence of symptoms. By the sixth month, the subjects had achieved an average of 8.8 of the pretreatment hierarchy items and 9 of the 12 had been able to take shopping trips alone to nearby cities.

This study is quite encouraging because it suggests that significant reductions in housebound agoraphobics' anxiety and avoidance behavior can be accomplished with minimal therapist contact. In these cases, the average contact time was only 7 hours per subject. Another recent study replicated these successful results and spent an average of only 3.5 hours in direct contact time.[8] This home-based, self-help approach to treating agoraphobia appears to be both effective and efficient.

I should note here that another recent attempt with a similar treatment program met with failure.[9] This study was similar in design, using a self-help manual for clients to work on their own to increase exposure to fear situations. The therapists maintained weekly phone contact to answer questions. However, in this latter study, in contrast to the two successful home-based programs, the therapists did not actively enlist or require a spouse or trusted companion to work closely with the clients. This element of having a helper to work with whoever provides motivation, support, and general assistance in working at difficult tasks is probably a critical element in agoraphobic treatment. After it became apparent that little progress was being made by the clients alone, these authors introduced therapists to participate actively in clients' exposure practice. With this added assistance, significant progress was made in five of the six clients. Thus, with the right combination of procedures and persons to assist and motivate, these treatments can be quite successful.

TREATMENT OF OBSESSIVE-COMPULSIVE DISORDER

Obsessive-compulsive disorders are perhaps the most treatment resistant of the anxiety disorders. The following case is illustrative of these difficulties. Although treatment was largely successful, the subject was not completely symptom free. The subject of this case study, which was reported by Robertson, Wendiggensen, and Kaplan, was 23 years old at the time treatment began and she had been diagnosed obsessive-compulsive since age 10.[10]

> At the time of treatment she had been virtually housebound for the past year and spent most of her time in bed occupied by her obsessive thoughts and compulsive rituals. Her obsessive thoughts centered on the fear that harm would come to her parents on whom she was totally dependent. To protect them from harm she engaged in superstitious rituals of counting and touching things a set number of times over and over. While performing these rituals she would utter to herself "good" thoughts in order to avoid intrusive "bad" thoughts. Her "good" thoughts consisted of self-deprecating statements while "bad" thoughts involved harm that might come to her parents.

As with most obsessive-compulsive disorders, the thoughts of harm led to an urge to conduct the compulsive rituals which, in turn, reduced the anxiety associated with the thoughts. The treatment approach then was to focus on breaking this sequence of events. First, response prevention was introduced, followed by attempts to disrupt the obsessive thoughts and restructure the client's maladaptive cognitions.

Before treatment began, there was a 10-day period in which the subject was allowed to become accustomed to the hospital setting in which the treatment was to be carried out. Also, pretreatment baseline data were gathered to assess the frequency of her thoughts and rituals. She was asked to record each occurrence of her motor rituals and obsessive thoughts. Initially, she reported an average of just under 400 motor rituals and just over 200 cognitive rituals per day.

The first treatment introduced was response prevention. The subject would be reminded and encouraged to resist carrying out her motor rituals of touching things over and over and to do so long enough to allow the experienced anxiety to decrease. This was highly effective in reducing the motor rituals to about 20 per day. However, with the decline of motor rituals came a sharp increase in cognitive rituals, up to nearly 400 per day.

To combat this increased cognitive activity, an exposure technique was introduced in which her bad thoughts were played to her over and over on a tape recording. Unfortunately, this exposure treatment was unsuccessful since the subject managed to avoid listening to the tape. Next, two cognitive procedures were introduced. A procedure called *systematic disruption* was used to interrupt her "good" thoughts which had kept out the "bad" thoughts. The therapists would contaminate her good thoughts by repeating to her the content from the bad thoughts. This procedure prevented her escaping from or avoiding the bad thoughts and allowed them to become habituated.

Concurrent with this disruption was the introduction of cognitive restructuring which focused on helping her see the senselessness of her fears that harm would come to her parents and the lack of necessity for her superstitious thinking. Also, the therapists worked at expanding her social activities and associations to reduce her dependence on her parents, which was seen as a large part of the source of her obsessive-compulsive behaviors. The tactics focusing on the cognitive activity resulted in a significant reduction in her cognitive rituals which decreased from about 400 to about 20 per day by the end of treatment.

Following treatment, there was still some level of cognitive and motor rituals being performed. However, these were no longer severe enough to impair her functioning. She was able to leave the hospital and, within six months, was working full time and living on her own. However, over time there was an increase in symptoms and after two years she was readmitted to the hospital for another treatment session.

The techniques used in the treatment of this case are those generally found most effective in reducing obsessive-compulsive behaviors. Response prevention focuses on the behavioral rituals while the cognitive disruptions and restructuring are aimed at changing the obsessional thoughts.

TREATMENT OF CHILDHOOD ANXIETY DISORDERS

A Childhood Posttraumatic Stress Disorder

Along with OCD, posttraumatic stress disorders are the most difficult anxiety disorders to treat. The following case described by Philip Saigh of the City University of New York details his treatment of a six and one-half-year-old Lebanese boy.[11]

> Joseph was referred for treatment by his school teacher due to an increasing inability to remember things, inability to attend, and frequent temper outbursts. His parents confirmed that at home he had similar difficulties, along with trauma-related recollections and nightmares, depression, and avoidance behavior. Twenty-five months prior, Joseph had been exposed to a bomb blast in which he witnessed others injured.

The treatment chosen for Joseph involved imaginal exposure of the traumatic scenes. The scenes included Joseph accompanied by his sister entering a shopping area, hearing a loud explosion followed by scenes of injured people, and of a man carrying an injured child. Before the actual treatment began, Joseph was given imagery training along with experience in relaxation. Once he was able to imagine these scenes clearly and had learned relaxation sufficiently, the flooding procedure was begun. This involved an initial 15-minute period of relaxation followed by 24 minutes of detailed visualization of the trauma scenes. By the end of 11 treatment sessions, Joseph was able to imagine 3 of the 4 trauma scenes with virtually no anxiety. The most difficult scene involving the injured child was somewhat more resistant but yet he managed to reduce his anxiety to this scene by 50 percent. Tested again 6 months later, he had maintained his gains. His general anxiety and depression levels had decreased, and his attention span increased. Imaginal exposure as applied in Joseph's case is also one of the effective components of treatment programs for adults with PTSD.

Posttraumatic stress disorder is one of the least understood of the anxiety disorders and one in which there is no agreed upon "best" treatment. However, many therapists would agree that some form of reexposure, as that used with Joseph, may be a necessary ingredient to successful treatment.

Separation Anxiety Disorder

The final treatment therapy to be described involved Joan, an 8-year-old child, who, since about the second grade, had refused to be left alone at home even for an instant. Even at the suggestion that her mother might step outside, Joan would become frightened and tearful. Lizette Peterson of the University of Missouri who conducted this case study and Joan's mother initially set the goal of having Joan able to stay in the house alone for a period of 10 minutes.[12]

The treatment began with teaching Joan some general

stress-management procedures that she was to use at the first signs of becoming fearful. These included muscle relaxation, deep breathing, and development of positive images that she could practice when negative images came to her. She also learned self-instructional training as a cognitive restructuring procedure, including self-statements as "I can handle it," which were to be used along with her positive images. Treatment proper involved Dr. Peterson and Joan's mother announcing that they would be leaving the house for progressively longer time periods until the 10-minute goal had been reached. At one point at Session 6, Joan had refused to participate at all. After some negotiation, she agreed to continue with the treatment and after successfully tolerating an 8-minute absence, Joan announced "the fear came and I made it go away" (p. 383). From that point on, her self-efficacy concerning her ability to stay alone remained high and she easily met her goal of staying alone for 10 minutes. This goal was achieved at Session 8. This success continued and Joan was then able to stay in her bedroom alone without parents close by and progressively able to stay home alone for longer and longer periods of time.

FEAR AND ANXIETY REDUCTION WITHOUT PROFESSIONAL INTERVENTION

Spontaneous Remission and Placebo Effects

Having just reviewed examples of some of the more effective methods for treating anxiety disorders, an important issue should be addressed: Do people with anxiety disorders require professional treatment? Can people overcome anxiety disorders on their own? These questions have been the subject of much debate and some research. I will briefly review two issues pertinent to this question. The first concerns *spontaneous remission* rates or the extent to which symptoms remit (go away) without professional treatment. The second issue concerns the effectiveness of self-help books or manuals in assisting persons to overcome anxiety and fears.

Nearly 40 years ago, Hans J. Eysenck of the University of London concluded that as many as two thirds of neurotic disorders (anxiety-based) get better in two years with or without treatment.[13] Although these figures have been disputed by some researchers, other recent evaluations of this area tend to concur with these figures.[14]

Whether Eysenck's two-thirds figure is correct or not, it is clear that a large proportion of persons with anxiety disorders do get better with or without treatment. Recall from Chapter 2 that as many as 90 percent of children develop some specific fear, and that these fears tend to dissipate with age, maturation, and increased experiences. Also, Agras found that among the clinical phobics identified in his 1969 community survey, virtually all of those under 20 years of age were greatly improved five years later.[15] Only 43 percent of those over 20 were so improved. Most recently, Barlow's anxiety disorders research group found in two studies of panic disorder that greater than one third of their control group who were placed on a waiting list were panic free in 12 weeks, even though they had not yet received treatment. In another group, 36 percent of those who had been given a placebo (an inactive substance) were panic free in 12 weeks.[16] Although we can expect that upward of one third of patients might get better without treatment, we should bear in mind that this one-third figure is considerably lower than the success rate of the cognitive behavioral treatment groups in these same studies. In these treatments, 85 to 87 percent were panic free in this same time period.

To investigate some of the possible reasons for untreated improvement, I conducted a survey of a group of people who had been previously fearful of spiders but, at the time of the survey, were tarantula enthusiasts.[17] Those who had overcome their spider fears attributed their improvement to the same factors included in the treatments described earlier: increased and accurate information, vicarious exposure to others who were not fearful (modeling), and various forms of exposure. For example, one previously fearful person related that a co-worker brought a terrarium containing a tarantula to the office. This unplanned exposure to tarantulas, along with information about them, eventually led not only to an elimination of the previous fear but to a strong liking and interest in them. However, I do not know how severe these fears were. It may be that milder, nonphobic fears are more subject to change under these informal "treatment" conditions than would be the case for more severe anxiety disorders. We do not have reliable information on spontaneous remission rates for all the different anxiety disorders and their degrees of severity, although there is a suggestion that obsessive-compulsive disorders are resistant to these effects.[18] We can conclude that between one half and two thirds of anxiety disorders may remit over a period of several years and one third may remit within a few weeks without formal treatment. However, much remains to be learned about the differential changes for each disorder type, age, severity, and the factors responsible for this change.

Self-Help Books

The second issue related to behavior change without professional intervention is the effectiveness of the plethora of self-help books found nowadays. Do they really work? The answer to this question, based on current research, is both yes and no. Unfortunately, most of the research on the effects of self-help books has been conducted on college students with milder or subclinical fears. In reviewing the research on these effects, Russell Glasgow and Gerald Rosen concluded that up to 50 percent of study participants report some positive effects from self-help manuals.[19] However, a major drawback in using these manuals is that 50 percent of the participants failed to complete the program as laid out. So, though there may be some positive effect from self-help books for some people, adherence to the program is a major problem.

For many people, and perhaps for most of those with severe problems, some therapist contact appears to be important. Recall that the self-help study of agoraphobics by Holden found virtually no effect when subjects were left on their own to complete a detailed program. However, when the therapists eventually became more actively involved, five of six subjects did show significant improvement. This was similar to the two home-based treatment programs described which included more therapist contact and had the assistance of a spouse.

At this stage of refinement of self-help manuals, I believe it is reasonable to conclude that some people, particularly those with milder anxiety conditions, can benefit without direct professional intervention. However, for more severe disorders such as agoraphobia and obsessive-compulsive disorder, some skilled professional intervention may be necessary, if even in an advisory capacity. Another alternative that is helping many today are the self-help groups.

Self-Help Groups

A number of highly popular self-help groups are now developing that offer both lay support and professional consultation. The Phobia Society of America has recently published a book to assist those who are interested in developing self-help groups. Information concerning this book, *Help Your Self: A Guide to Organizing a Phobia Self-Help Group,* can be obtained from:

> Phobia Society of America
> P. O. Box 2066
> Rockville, MD 20852-2066

In Great Britain, a group called Triumph Over Phobia (TOP), a self-treatment approach, has been developed by a former airplane phobic. This program is supervised by Isaac Marks of the Department of Psychiatry of the University of London, whose name has appeared frequently throughout this book. TOP uses an approach similar to that described by Barlow in that they follow Marks's book, *Living with Fear*, which describes fears and phobias and offers details of a self-help treatment program.[20]

A particularly useful self-help and information service is provided by a group in New Hampshire, headed by Avis McKenzie. Among the services that are provided is a newsletter for persons who have experienced anxiety disorders and depression. This newsletter, "Second Chance," can be obtained for an annual subscription of $22.00, by writing to:

> Second Chance
> Newsletter
> P. O. Box 627
> Rochester, NH 03867

Among the several features of the newsletter are interviews with individuals, descriptions of anxiety experiences, tips and procedures for dealing with anxiety, and learning to live without the debilitating effects of anxiety. An additional service is their pen-pal arrangement in which individuals may be placed in contact with others with whom they may correspond. This approach is an effective means of promoting camaraderie and social support during trying times. Finally, their hot line, call-in information service is a great boon to those in immediate need of general information on anxiety disorders, support groups, reading lists, and the like. Avis McKenzie reports that they now have numerous international contacts as well as many throughout North America. This service appears to have become an anxiety-disorders information clearinghouse.

SUMMARY AND CONCLUSIONS

The behavior therapy and cognitive behavior therapy procedures have been found highly effective for treating most anxiety disorders. The therapy procedures described in Chapter 8 and illustrated here focus on changing the three response components of fear and anxiety. They attempt to change the anxiety-producing thought processes, the avoidance and escape behavior that can serve to strengthen the fear, and the physiological reactivity that is so distressing and that can serve as cues to further anxiety responsiveness.

These treatments have been found to be highly effective for simple phobia, for panic disorder, and agoraphobia, with success rates approaching 100 percent in many studies.[21] Other disorders, such as OCD and PTSD, while amenable to treatment in greater than 50 percent of cases, are somewhat more resistant with present methods. But effective treatment here is advancing as well.

The success rates of the cognitive behavior therapies also compare very favorably to those achieved by drug treatments. In most studies that compare treatment effectiveness, the psychologically based treatments are found to be equal to or to exceed the effectiveness of drug treatments.[22,23] The drug treatments, which are to be described in the next chapter, do add an additional element to the overall anxiety disorders treatment armamentarium. In treatment resistant cases that often occur in OCD, for example, some new drugs can now help individuals whose condition was refractory to the cognitive behavioral treatments. Now that there is a range of both psychological and medical treatments with proven effectiveness, a large majority of patients with anxiety disorders need no longer suffer.[23]

REFERENCES

1. Ronald Kleinknecht and Douglas Bernstein, "Assessment of Dental Fear," *Behavior Therapy* 9 (1978): 626–634.
2. Lars-Goran Öst, "Behavioral Treatment of Thunder and Lightning Phobias, *Behaviour Research and Therapy* 16 (1978): 197–207.
3. C. K. Cohn, R. E. Kron, and J. P. Brady, "Single Case Study: A Case of Blood-Illness-Injury Phobia Treated Behaviorally," *Journal of Nervous and Mental Disease* 162 (1976): 65–68.
4. Elizabeth Klonoff, Jeffrey Janta, and Benjamin Kaufman, "The Use of Systematic Desensitization to Overcome Resistance to Magnetic Resonance Imaging (MRI) Scanning," *Journal of Behavior Therapy and Experimental Psychiatry* 17 (1986): 198–192.

5. M. Biran, F. Augusto, and G. T. Wilson, "In Vivo Exposure vs. Cognitive Restructuring in the Treatment of Scriptophobia," *Behaviour Research and Therapy* 19 (1981): 525–532.

6. Ronald M. Rapee, "A Case of Panic Disorder Treated with Breathing Retraining," *Journal of Behavior Therapy and Experimental Psychiatry* 16 (1985): 63–65.

7. Andrew Mathews, John Teasdale, M. Munby, D. Johnston, and P. Shaw, "A Home-Based Treatment Program for Agoraphobia," *Behavior Therapy* 8 (1977): 915–924.

8. L. Jannoun, M. Munby, J. Catalan, and M. Gelder, "A Home-Based Treatment Program for Agoraphobia: Replication and Controlled Evaluation, *Behavior Therapy* 11 (1980): 294–305.

9. A. E. Holden, Jr., Gerald T. O'Brien, David H. Barlow, D. Stetson, and A. Infantino, "Self-Help Manual for Agoraphobia: A Preliminary Report of Effectiveness," *Behavior Therapy* 14 (1983): 545–556.

10. J. Robertson, P. Wendiggensen, and I. Kaplan, "Towards a Comprehensive Treatment for Obsessional Thoughts," *Behaviour Research and Therapy* 21 (1983): 347–356.

11. Philip Saigh, "*In Vitro* Flooding in the Treatment of a 6-year-old Boy's Posttraumatic Stress Disorder," *Behaviour Research and Therapy* 24 (1986): 685–688.

12. Lizette Peterson, "Not Safe at Home: Behavioral Treatment of a Child's Fear of Being at Home Alone," *Behavior Therapy and Experimental Psychiatry* 18 (1987): 381–385.

13. Hans J. Eysenck, "The Effects of Psychotherapy: An Evaluation," *Journal of Consulting Psychology* 16 (1952): 319–324.

14. Stanley Rachman and G. T. Wilson, *The Effects of Psychological Therapy*, 2nd ed. (Oxford, England: Pergamon Press, 1980).

15. Stewart Agras, H. A. Chapin, and D. C. Oliveau, "The Natural History of Phobia," *Archives of General Psychiatry* 26 (1972): 315–317.

16. Janet Klosko, David Barlow, R. B. Tassinari, and Jerome Cerny, "A Comparison of Alprazolam and Cognitive-Behavior Therapy in Treatment of Panic Disorder," *Journal of Consulting and Clinical Psychology* 58 (1990): 77–84.

17. Ronald Kleinknecht, "The Origin and Remissions of Fear in a Group of Tarantula Enthusiasts," *Behaviour Research and Therapy* 20 (1982): 437–443.

18. Stanley Rachman and G. T. Wilson, *The Effects of Psychological Therapy*, 2nd ed. (Oxford, England: Pergamon Press, 1980).

19. Russell Glasgow and Gerald Rosen, "Behavioral Bibliotherapy: A Review of Self-Help Behavior Therapy Manuals," *Psychological Bulletin* 85 (1978): 1–23.

20. Isaac Marks, *Living with Fear* (New York: McGraw-Hill), 1978.

21. Thomas Borkovec, "Treatment of Anxiety Disorders: The State of the Art." Paper presented to the Third World Congress of Behavior Therapy, Edinburgh, 1988.

22. George Clum, "Psychological Interventions vs. Drugs in the Treatment of Panic Disorder," *Behavior Therapy* 20 (1989): 429–457.

23. Klosko *et al.*, "A Comparison of Alprazolam," 77–84.

Drug Treatment of Anxiety Disorders

Psychotropic drugs are probably the most common form of treatment for anxiety and anxiety disorders. However, they are not necessarily the most effective treatment for anxiety disorders. Their extensive use is due, in part, to the fact that one of the first places people go for help with anxiety problems is to their family physician. Most of the psychotherapeutic drug prescriptions are written by nonpsychiatric physicians who are not trained in the treatment procedures described in the previous two chapters, nor do they have the time to devote to the treatment of anxiety disorders. Many of these drugs provide rapid relief from anxiety and are useful and effective as a first step to dealing with anxiety and stress responses. Since they often relieve anxiety, the person may look no further for other treatments. These drugs, together with psychologically based treatments described previously, provide a wide array of treatment alternatives to those individuals who are suffering from anxiety, fear, and panic disorders.

In Chapters 8 and 9, the psychological treatments that were described were shown to be highly effective for many of the anxiety disorders. However, for some conditions, such as OCD and PTSD, psychological treatments are effective over the long term for only about 50 to 60 percent of patients. These treatments are either ineffective or offer only short-term relief for others. An alternative and adjunctive treatment for these disorders is the use of drugs or pharmacotherapy. Drug treatment can be effective in some cases where psychological treatments were unsuccessful or in which the therapeutic effect is needed more quickly. In other cases, the combination of drug treatment with psychological treatments may be more effective than either alone. Together, these treatment courses can help many anxiety-disordered patients today.

In this chapter, then, the drugs most commonly used to treat each of the anxiety disorders will be described and their effectiveness will be evaluated. To comprehend more fully these drug effects, a summary of how these drugs exert their anxiety-reducing effects is provided.

In recent years, psychotherapeutic drugs increasingly have been used in the treatment of psychological disorders. The national survey conducted by Uhlenhuth and his colleagues in 1983 found that 16 percent of the adult population in the United States had used one form of psychotherapeutic drug within the year prior to the survey. The most commonly used drugs, those most relevant to this book, are identified as *antianxiety agents* or *anxiolytics* and were being used by 11 percent of the sample.

HOW DRUGS AFFECT MOOD AND BEHAVIOR

The *psychotropic* or *psychotherapeutic* drugs exert their influence on mood and behavior by altering communication channels among nerve cells in the brain. At this point, all of the complicated chemical processes are not fully understood. Nonetheless, a sufficient amount is known to help us understand some of the basic processes by which taking a pill can translate into feeling and behaving differently and, in our specific case, can reduce fear and anxiety.

First, it is important to realize that the brain is made up of virtually billions of tiny nerve cells called *neurons*. Bundles of neurons make up nerves. Information that travels about the brain does so through these neurons by way of electrical impulses. This network of neurons and their electrical impulses work similarly to the way telephone wires take information from one phone and, through various connections, deliver it where the caller wanted it to go. What we experience as feeling, thinking, and behavior derives from the communication among these neurons of the brain. Thus, the critical point is understanding how neurons communicate with each other and how alterations of these communication processes can, in turn, alter our mental experience.

Understanding the communication process is the most critical aspect of understanding how drugs work. Although neurons must interact with other neurons, they are not physically connected like electrical wires. Between each neuron there is a minuscule gap called a *synapse*. For neurons to "communicate" with one another, chemicals are secreted that bridge the synaptic gap. If we begin with a neuron that is electrically stimulated, it can be seen carrying an electrical charge down its length until it reaches the synapse. At the end or terminal point of this neuron, chemicals are stored. When the electrical impulse reaches these chemicals, it causes them to be released into the synapse. These communicating chemicals (several of which are to be described later), are called *neurotransmitters*. On the other side of the synapse is another neuron and on its surface are the chemical *receptor* sites—tiny places where certain chemicals, neurotransmitters, of specific molecular shape can lock into, similar to the way a key fits into a lock. When enough of a specific neurotransmitter locks into the corresponding receptors, it activates this neuron to create a continuation of the electrical impulse onto yet other neurons. Thus, a chain of electrical information is transmitted throughout the brain. The psychotropic drugs exert their effects on mood and behavior by altering the availability and activity of the neurotransmitter chemicals. This, in turn, alters the transmission of information throughout the brain or through specific areas of the brain that depend on that particular neurotransmitter for communication.

Before we move on to further elaboration of this communication process, one more process that affects drug effects has to be described. When the neurotransmitter chemical has been released, has crossed the synapses, has locked into the receptor site, and has stimulated activity in the new neuron, it then is released from the activated neuron. After being released from the receptor site, the neurotransmitter is either chemically broken down into smaller molecules or is taken back into the terminal neuron from which it was originally released. This process of taking back the chemical into the releasing neuron is called *reuptake*. These processes are critically important because if the neurotransmitter is left free in the synapse, it can continue to stimulate the neuron. As we will see, alteration of these two processes of reuptake or breakdown by other chemicals (drugs) will affect brain function and will thus alter how one thinks and feels.

The basic elements of nerve transmission provide a picture of how drugs affect us. However, there are a few more details that need to be described to understand more adequately how the different drugs operate on the different aspects of anxiety. First, there are several chemical substances that serve as neurotransmitters in the brain. Some neurons are affected by one transmitter, but not by others. Also, a particular set of nerves or pathways may affect one set of psychological disorders, such as anxiety, and all the neurons in the specific nerve pathway will use the same neurotransmitter. Thus, any alteration of this transmitter substance in the brain will affect all nerve transmission in this anxiety tract. Furthermore, when some neurotransmitter substances fill a neuron's receptors, it causes or facilitates the neuron to "fire" or become "excited" and thus sends an impulse on to the next neuron. Of course, these processes are important so that information can get around. However, nerves cannot just fire all of the time or the brain would be in a continuous state of "excitation," which would be analogous to a car with the accelerator depressed and no brakes. Thus, to provide a necessary balance in the nervous system, nature has provided a system of brakes in the form of "inhibitory" transmitter systems. When some neurotransmitters fill the receptor sites, they prevent or inhibit the neuron from firing or sending further information. These two types of systems, excitatory and inhibitory, work in concert under normal circumstances to provide a check-and-balance system that keeps the brain and our mental processes under control. Any alteration of these systems results in changes in mood and behavior. When these systems are not functioning in a balanced way because of stresses or perhaps because of one's inherited characteristics, the psychotherapeutic drugs can alter the neurochemical functions and thus restore the person to a more balanced or relaxed state. Next, we turn to the specific drugs that are used to treat anxiety disorders.

PSYCHOTROPIC DRUGS FOR THE ANXIETY DISORDERS

In this section, I will describe some of the drugs that are used in the treatment of anxiety disorders, the research concerning the effectiveness of these drugs, and some of the postulated mechanisms that are thought to be responsible for their effects. Although many of these drugs have been shown to be useful in treating some anxiety disorders, it should be noted that exact biochemical mechanisms through which they exert their effects are currently unknown. Also, it is important to realize that drugs, as they affect the neurotransmitter systems, do not selectively affect only the single psychological function that is desired. Rather, they affect a variety of other bodily functions that use the same neurotransmitter, which is why we get side effects. Side effects represent drug action on other bodily systems that also use the neurotransmitter that is being altered. For example, dry mouth is a common side effect of the tricyclic antidepressants, which as we will see also have antipanic effects. These drugs are aimed at affecting certain neurotransmitter systems in the brain. However, because the drug is transported through the bloodstream, it is taken to all parts of the body. Any part of the nervous system that can be reached by the drug is affected; consequently, since neurons controlling saliva are affected by these drugs, one gets a dry mouth.

The three classes of drugs to be described are (1) the anti-anxiety agents (sometimes called *minor tranquilizers*) (2) the *beta-adrenergic blocking agents* (beta-blockers), and (3) the *antidepressants*. Some of the antidepressants, while alleviating depression in many people, also affect some anxiety functions, particularly panic and are thus sometimes referred to as *antipanic* drugs.

The Antianxiety Agents

The Benzodiazepines

The class of antianxiety drugs most widely used in anxiety disorders are the *benzodiazepines*. These drugs include a variety of related compounds. All have similar antianxiety effects but vary from each other in terms of potency and length of time they exert their effects. Among the most widely used of the benzodiazepines are diazepam (Valium), chlordiazepoxide (Librium), and alprazolam (Xanax). Other drugs within this class are shown in Table 13.

The benzodiazepines were introduced to the U.S. phar-

TABLE 13
Antianxiety Drugs

Generic name	Trade name
The benzodiazepines	
Alprazolam	Xanax
Chlordiazepoxide	Librium
Chlorazepate	Tranxene
Diazepam	Valium
Lorazepam	Avitan
Oxazepam	Serax
Triazolam	Halcion
Nonbenzodiazepines	
Buspirone	BuSpar
Beta blocker	
Propranolol	Inderol

maceutical market in the early 1960s (Librium, 1960, Valium, 1962) and immediately became extremely popular among prescribing physicians and patients and ultimately became one of the most widely used prescription drugs in the world. By 1973, Valium was the single most prescribed drug in the United States and Librium was third.[1] Part of the popularity of these drugs was due to the variety of conditions for which they appeared useful. In addition to treating anxiety states for which they are most commonly prescribed, they are used as skeletal muscle relaxants, as epilepsy control agents, in anesthesia, and as presurgical medication. However, it is tension and anxiety-related problems that account for the majority of prescriptions. As has been noted throughout this book, anxiety is perhaps the most prevalent of all psychological symptoms and the base for the most prevalent of the psychological disorders.

These drugs affect anxiety through their action as general central nervous system depressants. That is, they tend to reduce the excitability of neurons and therefore slow many brain functions. After taking these drugs, the anxious individual experiences physical and mental calmness, a reduction in felt tension, greater ease in falling to sleep, a general feeling of well-being, and often a feeling of being better able to cope with the stresses in their lives.

For most people, these effects are quite immediate and dramatic. However, these anxiety-reducing effects have been likened to the effect of aspirin on fever.[2] Aspirin clearly reduces the fever, but does nothing for the cause of the fever. Both are generalized treatments of symptoms. Of course, this is true of all psychotherapeutic drugs. They do not cure the problem.[3] They only make the person feel better while the drug is active in the body.

Numerous clinical and experimental studies have documented the anxiety-reducing effects of the various benzodiazepines.[4,5] In particular, many authorities suggest that they are most effective in reducing generalized anxiety disorder and various forms of anticipatory anxiety.[6,7] In contrast, some reports indicate that the benzodiazepines were not particularly effective in treating panic attacks in agoraphobia or panic disorder.[8,9]

However, it now seems clearer that at least some of the benzodiazepines may indeed reduce panic attacks as well as more generalized anxiety. Noyes and colleagues found diazepam (Valium) to be equally effective in reducing panic disorder, agoraphobia, and generalized anxiety disorder.[10] Similar results were obtained using alprazolam (Xanax), a newer, high-potency benzodiazepine.[11] In recent years, Xanax has become quite popular because it was found to be effective in treating the anxiety component of agoraphobia as well as the accompanying depression. However, even though Xanax has been shown to have relatively quick treatment effects for some people, a recent large-scale study of its effectiveness has shown that just over 50 percent of the patients were panic-free after two months.[12] While this and related drugs are clearly useful in reducing anxiety and panic for many, they are not panaceas.

Thus far, these antianxiety agents do not appear by themselves to be effective treatments of obsessive-compulsive disorders nor are they effective for simple phobias. However, there are clinical reports that they can be useful adjuncts in the treatment of phobias. For example, Joseph Wolpe, originator of systematic desensitization, reported a case in which he used Valium to assist in the treatment of agoraphobia.[13] The drug was administered to enable the patient to begin a graduated exposure treatment. With Valium, the patient was able to venture alone from home and to drive. Once this treatment was established, the dosage was decreased until he was eventually able to manage these situations in a drug-free state. The antianxiety drugs appear to offer some beneficial effects for anxiety disorders, both when used alone for generalized anxiety, for panic attacks, and agoraphobia, and when used as part of an exposure treatment.

How They Work

The possible neural or brain areas through which these antianxiety drugs might affect panic was described in Chapter 5 in the context of Gorman's neurophysiological theory of anxiety disorders. You may recall that they postulated the limbic system as the area that maintained and was largely responsible for anticipatory anxiety. And this area, in turn, could influence the brain stem areas such as the locus coeruleus, the areas that seemed most responsible for panic. Thus, if the anticipatory anxiety were quelled by the benzodiazepines, it could not build up to stimulate panic attacks. Thus, there could be an effect of the benzodiazepines on panic, operating indirectly on the more specific panic-generating centers in the brain stem.

The physical and psychological effects of these drugs appear to come from generally calming and tension-reduction properties rather than from specific action affecting designated symptoms; that is, they are not antipanic drugs. It appears that they reduce the general excitability of persons, which, in turn, may allow them to gain exposure to the feared situations.

The specific biochemical mechanism by which these drugs exert their calming effects has become the subject of considerable research and theorizing. One proposed mechanism is that the benzodiazepines facilitate some naturally occurring neural inhibitory processes in the brain. It is believed that they interact with and facilitate the effects of gamma-aminobutyric acid (GABA) a neurotransmitter. GABA is one of those neurotransmitters that serve to inhibit nerve transmission. For example, when the neuron in which GABA is the chemical transmitter is stimulated and GABA is released across the synapse and binds with the receptor on the adjacent neuron, it decreases the chance of the next neuron continuing the transmission. This is referred to as the braking system. The benzodiazepines can also attach to some of the GABA receptors and when they do, they assist GABA in increasing the neural inhibition, thus rendering certain parts of the brain less excitable. Therefore, the person is less likely to react to situations with anxiety or fear.[14]

Adverse Side Effects

Although these antianxiety drugs are useful in treating some of the anxiety disorders, they are not without drawbacks. Although these drugs block nerve transmission having to do with anxiety, they not only affect anxiety-related brain centers but are also general neural depressants that affect other brain functions as well. For example, some of the potentially more negative side effects of this neural inhibition include decreased psychomotor coordination and cognitive functioning.[15] Patients taking these drugs are cautioned by their prescribing physicians that it may be hazardous to operate dangerous machinery or to drive while taking the benzodiazepines.

A further and potentially serious problem is that long-term use of these agents can develop into a physical dependency. Abrupt withdrawal from these drugs can result in a rebound effect in which anxiety is increased over predrug levels and withdrawal symptoms can be experienced, such as insomnia, nausea, and stomach cramps.[16] More recently, some reports have appeared showing that abrupt discontinuation of these drugs can cause seizures in some individuals.[17]

Buspirone

The most recent of the antianxiety drugs is buspirone (Bu-Spar), which is chemically different from the benzodiazepines. This new drug also differs from the others in that it does not appear to exert the many negative side effects previously mentioned. In a series of studies, BuSpar was found to cause less drowsiness, sedation, and fatigue, and to impair motor function less. Also, in contrast with the benzodiazepines, BuSpar does not interact with alcohol. That is, when alcohol was taken in combination with, say, Valium, a person's impairment became greater than when taking either drug individually. BuSpar does not seem to cause impairment on its own nor does it enhance alcohol's adverse effects on performance.[18]

Another major difference between buspirone and the benzodiazepines is that the person does not experience an immediate calming effect. With such drugs as Valium or Xanax, the sedating and calming drug effect can be felt within a few minutes. With BuSpar, the calming effect comes on more gradually, over a period of days. Thus, it is believed that this drug will not be subject to abuse as has often been the case with the benzodiazepines because of their immediate and powerful calming effects. Furthermore, prolonged buspirone use does not create a physical dependence; neither withdrawal nor overdose is lethal; the person just becomes ill.[19] Thus, buspirone appears to be much safer than the other agents although since it is relatively new, much remains to be learned about its possible uses and effects in a clinical setting.

The Antidepressants

Antidepressants are the second class of drugs used in treating anxiety disorders. Although they were developed for and are highly effective in the treatment of depression, some of these drugs have also been shown to be useful for certain of the anxiety disorders, particularly panic disorder and obsessive-compulsive disorder. The drugs most effective for each disorder will be described in turn.

Antipanic Effects

There are two subclassifications of antidepressants, both of which contain drugs that are capable of reducing panics. These include the *monoamine oxidase inhibitors* (MAO-I) and the *tricyclic* compounds. Examples of each of these types of drugs are listed in Table 14.

Several of the so-called antidepressants, such as imipramine, have satisfactorily demonstrated antipanic effects. These drugs appear to have their major effect on reducing more or less "spontaneous" panic attacks, those that seem not to be associated with specific feared or dangerous stimuli. Some researchers believe that these drugs are highly specific to panic reduction and have virtually no effect on more general or anticipatory anxiety.[20] Others are not in full agreement, because they believe that these drugs can affect all types of anxiety. Nonetheless, there is little debate over the antipanic effects. Panic-disordered patients taking these drugs often describe feeling a panic

TABLE 14
Antidepressants Used for Anxiety Disorders

	Generic name	Trade name
Monoamine oxidase inhibitors as antipanic drugs	Isocarboxazid	Marplan
	Phenelzine	Nardil
Tricyclics as antipanic drugs	Imipramine	Tofranil
	Desipramine	Norpramin
	Amitriptyline	Elavil
	Nortriptyline	Aventyl
	Doxepin	Sinequan
Tricyclics as antiobsessive drugs	Clomipramine	Anafranil
	Fluoxetine	Prozac

attack coming on with increasing heart rate and the like, but, surprisingly, they find that the attack just does not escalate to its usual peak; it just trails off and diminishes, leaving the person pleasantly puzzled. These antipanic effects do not occur immediately upon taking the drugs. One cannot take one of these drugs when an attack is coming on and expect it to help, as might be done with the benzodiazepines. Rather, it may take up to several weeks for the full antipanic effects to reach maximum. In this way, antidepressants are more like BuSpar.

In agoraphobic cases, where both panic and anticipatory anxiety are major components, some investigators recommend using antidepressants to reduce the panic attacks along with a benzodiazepine to reduce the generalized, anticipatory anxiety.[21] However, others suggest that if these drugs are used, it is reasonable to administer antidepressants to diminish the panic effects and to use such behavioral treatments as exposure to reduce the agoraphobic avoidance. Yet others, including David Barlow and his colleagues, point out that their research has demonstrated that cognitive and behavioral treatment programs, like the one his group has developed, are effective in combating both panic and anticipatory anxiety. And their latest study has shown that these treatments are more effective than some drug treatments incorporating Xanax.[22] In any event, with this variety of treatments, both psychological and pharmacological, the majority of persons with panic disorder and agoraphobia can be treated successfully.

Many of the antidepressants shown in Table 14 have also been reported to be at least partially successful in treating post-traumatic stress disorder in combat veterans. However, none of these drugs has been found to be universally successful with PTSD patients and only a minority of patients are significantly helped. Thus, PTSD remains one anxiety disorder that is yet in search of a widely successful treatment, whether psychological or chemical.

Antiobsessive Effects

One of the more significant breakthroughs in recent years in the treatment of anxiety disorders has been the discovery of a successful, although limited, drug treatment for obsessive-compulsive disorder. Two of the newer tricyclic antidepressant compounds have been found to significantly diminish obsessive ruminations and compulsive behavioral rituals. These drugs have been found to be effective in treating some obsessive-compulsive patients who were not responsive to other treatments, such as response prevention, which was described in Chapters 8 and 9. One of these drugs, Anafranil, has been shown in a recent study to reduce substantially symptoms in 58 percent of obsessive-compulsive patients.[23]

As with the antipanic drugs, it is not known just how this process acts to reduce obsessive thoughts and compulsive behaviors. Although the figure of helping only 58 percent of patients may not seem too successful, it is as good or better than any other known treatment to date. Since some OCD patients who do not respond positively to behavioral treatments (such as response prevention), do respond to these drugs, there is thus an expanded number of treatments available for them.

How They Work

Several attempts have been made to explain how anti-depressant drugs, originally developed for treating depression, can also treat panics and OCD. One suggestion is that they exert their effects by treating a depression which is so often found to coexist in panic disorder and OCD patients. This would assume that these anxiety disorders are manifestations of depression.[24,25] However, today, most researchers believe that the antianxiety effect is not due to reduced depression but to some more specific effect on the mechanisms that cause panic attacks or obsessive symptoms. Indeed, it has been proposed that the antidepressants may not be effective for treating anxious persons who are also severely depressed.[26,27]

Although the mechanism by which these drugs affect anxiety disorders is not precisely known, there is increasing evidence (see Chapter 5) that some of these drugs affect the locus coeruleus, which is the brain-stem center that is intimately involved in the generation of panics. Further, it has been hypothesized that, as with the benzodiazepines, the GABA (inhibitory), neurotransmitter systems are involved.[28] The antipanic effects of these drugs is thought to stem from their effect on the norepinephrine neurotransmitter systems. Although the tricyclics and the MAO-inhibitors work somewhat differently, the net effect of both is to leave more of the neurotransmitter available at the synapse.

The antiobsessive effects of Anafranil and Prozac seem to be operating through their effects of selectively inhibiting the reuptake of the neurotransmitter *serotonin*, which would leave more of it available for nerve transmission. Precisely how leaving more serotonin available in the synapse leads to a lessening of obsessive or compulsive behavior is, of course, still a mystery. This neurotransmitter is also thought to be involved in some forms of depression as well in OCD. While the search goes on for a better understanding of how these drugs exert their antianxiety effects, the patients for whom other treatments have been unsuccessful are fortunate to have them at their disposal.

Side Effects

As with the antianxiety drugs, the antidepressants also have unpleasant side effects. In studies by Zitrin, who investigated the anxiety-reducing effects, as many as 29 percent of the subjects dropped out of therapy because of difficulties from the side effects.[29] Others found even greater percentages of dropouts, some over 40 percent.[30] Foremost among the side effects are blurred vision, dizziness, drowsiness, dry mouth, weight gain, and nervousness. Because of these side effects and since the cognitive behavior therapy procedures are successful in treating phobias and panic attacks, Zitrin recommended that these drugs be used only in those cases that have not responded to psychological treatment.[31] As a consequence, this proposes a two-tiered procedure for treatment. First, it would seem reasonable to try the behavioral or cognitive behavior treatments. If these are less than fully successful, one of the antidepressants can be introduced to further enhance treatment effects.

The Beta Blockers

Of those drugs that are used for treating some anxiety disorders, the third class is quite different from the two previously described. The beta blockers do not exert their effects directly by altering brain neurons. Rather, they block the transmission of certain peripheral, as opposed to central (brain), nerves that compose portions of the sympathetic nervous system. The neurons that they selectively block are those that use the transmitter adrenaline or epinephrine. Adrenaline is the neurotransmitter that stimulates the nerves that directly affect the heart muscle. Thus, these drugs directly block the nerves that stimulate the heart to beat faster. These drugs have been observed to block the rapid heart rate and increased blood pressure experienced during intense anxiety or panic attacks. The beta blockers, such as propranolol (Inderol), appeared to hold great promise as yet another drug which could effectively treat anxiety disorders.

Noyes and his colleagues performed a series of studies to

evaluate these drugs. Although he found them to reduce the physiological component of anxiety, they appeared to have little or no effect on the cognitive component. In a trial comparing the effects of propranolol to Valium, he reported that propranolol was the superior treatment for chronically anxious patients whose primary response was physiological, whereas Valium was superior for patients whose primary symptoms were psychological or cognitive anxiety.

However, this matter of different drugs for different manifestations of anxiety is far from settled. In another study, Noyes and his colleagues compared the effects of Valium and propranolol on a group of patients with panic disorder, agoraphobia, and generalized anxiety disorder. They found Valium to be highly effective for 20 of 21 patients, whereas propranolol resulted in improvement in only 10 of 21 patients.[32] Further, Valium was more effective than propranolol in reducing both the physiological reactions of the panic attacks and the cognitive components.

One area that has shown some promise for beta blockers is with musicians. Several studies have shown that musicians taking the beta blocker Inderol report less anxiety while performing compared with placebo. However, these subjects were not clinically anxious and had not sought treatment; they were experiencing more normal anxiety. The effect for them was presumably a reduction in normal anxiety-related heart rate that may have been sufficient to cause some interference with their performance. Others suggest that even though this effect may be shown initially, the effect does not persist for future performances. Thus far, these drugs have not been found to be widely effective with persons with true anxiety disorders, although they may help some people with lower levels of anxiety.

SUMMARY AND CONCLUSIONS

Drug treatment for the anxiety disorders continues to show promising results. Further development of safe and effective treatments is still needed for some of the more refractory anxiety disorders such as OCD. While some highly positive effects have been reported for all three classes of drugs, there are some problems that remain to be overcome. First, many patients drop out of treatment due to intolerable, although not damaging, side effects such as dry mouth, drowsiness, and dizziness. Also, while drugs such as Xanax may be effective only in about 50 percent of cases, the clinician must weigh the possible benefits against the risk of abuse and possible physical dependence. Judicious use of these drugs, however, may aid many patients. Zitrin's recommendation of using cognitive behavior therapy procedures as the first treatment of choice would seem to have considerable merit. His alternative is especially attractive in light of the recent study by Janet Klosko and David Barlow in which 86 percent of patients receiving the cognitive behavioral treatment were panic free following treatment compared with the 50 percent success rate for those receiving Xanax. However, for those cases in which psychological approaches alone do not appear sufficient, or for which more rapid results are necessary, an appropriate drug treatment is available.

REFERENCES

1. Barry Blackwell, "Psychotropic Drugs in Use Today: The Role of Diazepam in Medical Procedure," *Journal of the American Medical Association* 125 (1973): 1637–1641.
2. Marvin E. Licky and Barbara Gordon, *Drugs for Mental Illness: A Revolution in Psychiatry* (New York: W. H. Freeman, (1983).
3. Karl Rickels, R. W. Downing, and A. Winoker, "Antianxiety Drugs: Clinical Use in Psychiatry," in *Handbook of Psychopharmacology: Vol. 13, Biology of Mood and Antianxiety Drugs,* L. L. Iverson, S. D. Iverson, and S. H. Snyder, ed. (New York: Plenum, 1978), 395–430.
4. Donald Klein, Rachel Gittelman, F. Quitkin, and A. Rifkin, *Diagnosis and Drug Treatment of Psychiatric Disorders: Adults and Children,* 2nd ed. (Baltimore: Williams & Wilkins, 1980).
5. D. J. Greenblatt and R. I. Shader, *Benzodiazepines in Clinical Practice* (New York: Raven Press, 1972).
6. Klein et al., *Diagnosis and Drug Treatment.*
7. Rickels et al., "Antianxiety Drugs," 395–430.

8. Ibid.

9. Klein et al., *Diagnosis and Drug Treatment*.

10. Russell Noyes, Jr., D. J. Anderson, J. Clancy, Raymond Crowe, D. J. Slyman, M. M. Ghonein, and J. V. Hinrichs, "Diazepam and Propranolol in Panic Disorder and Agoraphobia," *Archives of General Psychiatry,* 41 (1984): 287–292.

11. G. Chauinard, L. Annable, R. Fontaine, and L. Solyom, "Alprazolam in the Treatment of Generalized Anxiety and Panic Disorders: A Double-Blind Placebo-Controlled Study," *Psychopharmacology* 77 (1982): 229–233.

12. James Ballenger, G. Burrows, R. DuPont, I. Lesser, R. Noyes, J. Pecknold, A. Riskin, and R. Swanson, "Alprazolam in Panic Disorder: Results from a Multicenter Trial: 1. Efficacy in Short Term Treatment," *Archives of General Psychiatry* 45 (1988): 413–422.

13. Joseph Wolpe, *The Practice of Behavior Therapy* (Oxford, England: Pergamon Press, 1973).

14. Marvin E. Licky, and Barbara Gordon, *Drugs for Mental Illness: A Revolution in Psychiatry* (New York: W. H. Freeman, (1983).

15. Ronald Kleinknecht and David Donaldson, "A Review of the Effects of Diazepam on Cognitive and Psychomotor Performance," *Journal of Nervous and Mental Disease* 161 (1975): 399–411.

16. R. Fontaine, L. Annable, P. Deaudry, P. Mercier, and G. Chouinard, "Efficacy and Withdrawal of Two Potent Benzodiabepines: Bromazepam and Lorazepam," *Psychopharmacology Bulletin* 21 (1985): 91–92.

17. M. Dhyanne Warner, Cecilia Peabody, Nashaat Boutros, and Harvey Whiteford, "Alprazolam and Withdrawal Seizures," *Journal of Nervous and Mental Disease* 178 (1990): 208–209.

18. Truman Schnable, Jr., "Evaluation of the Safety and Side Effect of Anxiety Agents," *American Journal of Medicine* 82 (Supplement 5A, 1987): 7–13.

19. Malcolm Lader, "Assessing the Potential for Buspirone Dependence or Abuse and Effects of Its Withdrawal," *American Journal of Medicine* 82 (Supplement 5A, 1987): 20–26.

20. Donald Klein, Donald Ross, and Patricia Cohen, "Panic and Avoidance in Agoraphobia: Application of Path Analysis to Treatment Studies," *Archives of General Psychiatry* 44 (1987): 377–385.

21. Desmond Kelly, *Anxiety and Emotions: Physiological Basis and Treatment,* (Springfield, Ill.: Charles Thomas, 1980).

22. Janet Klosko, David Barlow, R. B. Tassinari, and Jerome Cerny, "A Comparison of Alprazolam and Cognitive-Behavior Therapy in Treatment of Panic Disorder," *Journal of Consulting and Clinical Psychology* 58 (1990): 77–84.

23. CIBA-GEIGY Corporation (Summit, New Jersey, 1990).

24. Isaac Marks, S. Gray, D. Cohen, R. Hill, D. Mawson, E. Ramm, and Richard Stern, "Imipramine and Brief Therapist Aided Exposure in Agoraphobics Having Self-Exposure Homework," *Archives of General Psychiatry* 40 (1983): 153–162.

25. Richard Stern and Isaac Marks, "Brief and Prolonged Flooding: A Comparison in Agoraphobic Patients," *Archives of General Psychiatry* 28 (1973): 270–276.
26. Desmond Kelly, *Anxiety and Emotions: Physiological Basis and Treatment*, (Springfield, Ill.: Charles Thomas, 1980).
27. Charlotte Zitrin, "Differential Treatment of Phobias: Use of Imipramine for Panic Attacks," *Journal of Behavior Therapy and Experimental Psychiatry* 14 (1983): 11–18.
28. David Sheehan, James Ballenger, and G. Jacobsen, "Treatment of Endogenous Anxiety with Phobic, Hysterical and Hypochondriacal Symptoms," *Archives of General Psychiatry* 37 (1980): 51–59.
29. Zitrin, "Differential Treatment," 11–18.
30. David Barlow, *Anxiety and Its Disorders*, (New York: Guilford Press, 1988).
31. Zitrin, "Differential Treatment," 11–18.
32. Russell Noyes, Jr., D. J. Anderson, J. Clancy, R. R. Crowe, D. J. Slyman, M. M. Ghonein, and J. V. Hinrichs, "Diazepam and Propranolol in Panic Disorder and Agoraphobia," *Archives of General Psychiatry* 41 (1984): 287–292.

Index